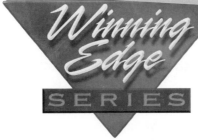

Aerobic Dance Exercise

DIXIE STANFORTH, M.S.
Lecturer, Department of Kinesiology and Health Education
The University of Texas
Austin, Texas
Fitness Editor, *Shape* Magazine
Contributing Editor, *Living Fit* Magazine

DEBORAH ELLISON, R.P.T.
Physical Therapist, specializing in ergonomics and women's health
Aerobic Dance Exercise Instructor
Program Design Consultant, Reebok
Editorial Board Member,
Fitness Matters of the American Council on Exercise

SERIES EDITOR
SCOTT O. ROBERTS, PH.D.
Department of Health, Physical Education, and Recreation
Texas Tech University
Lubbock, Texas

McGraw-Hill

**New York San Francisco Washington, D.C. Auckland Bogotá
Caracas Lisbon London Madrid Mexico City Milan
Montreal New Delhi San Juan Singapore
Sydney Tokyo Toronto**

McGraw-Hill

A Division of The McGraw·Hill Companies

Vice President and Publisher: James M. Smith
Senior Acquisitions Editor: Vicki Malinee
Developmental Editor: Brian Morovitz
Project Manager: Gayle Morris
Manuscript Editing: AlphaByte & Co.
Designer: David Zielinski
Manufacturing Manager: Betty Richmond
Cover Photographer: Bill Leslie
Series Photographer: James Crnkovich

NOTE: Not all exercises are suitable for everyone. To reduce the risk of injury in your case, consult your doctor before beginning this or any exercise program. The instructions and advice presented are not intended as a substitute for medical counseling.

Printed in the United States of America
Composition by DocuComp Services
Lithography by Accu-Color Inc.
Printing/binding by R.R. Donnelly, Inc.

Mosby–Year Book, Inc.
11830 Westline Industrial Drive
St. Louis, Missouri 63146

International Standard Book Number: 0-8151-8143-4

99 00 / 9 8 7 6 5 4 3 2

PREFACE

Most people do not exercise, so we congratulate you on your choice, whether you are just starting a program or have exercised for years. You have probably chosen to exercise for various reasons. You may want to lose some weight. You may want to reduce stress. You may simply want to feel better and have more energy. Exercise can help you do all that and more!

Aerobic dance is a fun way to get fit and stay fit. *Aerobic Dance Exercise* is designed to help you develop healthy attitudes about your body, educate you about the role of diet and exercise in developing and maintaining fitness, and at the same time teach you safe and effective dance exercise techniques.

▶ Audience

This text is designed for anyone interested in developing a personal fitness program, as well as students in academic courses on aerobic dance exercise, which are extremely popular today. The book is intended to be be an easy-to-read, useful tool that provides information on how to get the most from your exercise program.

▶ Features

The information in this text is material you will use for the rest of your life because it contains basic lifestyle lessons on everything from making wise dietary choices to optimal posture for sitting, standing, or dancing. Chapter 1, Introduction to Aerobic Dance Exercise, details the evolution of aerobic exercise and provides detailed information on high- and low-impact classes, step aerobics, and slide training. Chapter 2 then lets you discover the "Big Picture" of fitness and how to develop a lifestyle that incorporates all of the components of fitness. In this text, you will learn about exercise progressions and different techniques used in aerobic dance exercise. Specific exercises as well as modifications to increase or decrease intensity will help you design workouts that are tailored to meet your needs and goals.

In addition, there are special features throughout the text that enhance its utility:

- Professional studio photographs illustrate proper techniques and modifications common to most aerobic classes.
- Each chapter has a bulleted list of objectives and closing summary that outline and reinforce the major points covered.
- Key words and terms have been made boldface and defined in the text. This will enable you to build a working vocabulary of concepts and principles necessary for understanding, beginning, and maintaining a physical fitness program.

- Special Fitness Tip boxes outline safety-related concepts, applications, and procedures for quick reference.
- Self-Assessments appear throughout the text to assist you in determining and tracking your fitness level. If you are using this text in a course, these assessments are perforated so you can hand them in as class assignments.
- Appendix A provides important tips on how to choose a quality aerobic fitness instructor.

▶ Ancillaries

To facilitate use of this text in the classroom, a printed Test Bank of approximately 150 questions is available to instructors. These questions, ranging from matching and true/false to brief-answer formats, allow for quick assessment of the basic rules and principles. Please contact your sales representative for additional information.

▶ Acknowledgements

We would like to thank the following reviewers who provided us with expert commentary during the development of this text:

Susan P. Backus, M.S.
Arkansas State University, Beebe

Bonnie K. Nygard, M.Ed.
University of Alaska, Anchorage

Jeannean Ryman, M.S.
University of Texas-Pan American

Julia Spresser, Ed.D.
Pittsburg State University

We would also like to thank Phil Stanforth, M.S., from the University of Texas-Austin, who read the manuscript numerous times and provided valuable contributions.

—Dixie Stanforth
Deborah Ellison

CONTENTS

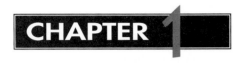

CHAPTER 1

INTRODUCTION TO AEROBIC DANCE EXERCISE

OBJECTIVES

After reading this chapter, you should be able to do the following:

- Discuss the difference between aerobic activity and aerobic dance exercise.
- Outline the evolution of aerobic dance exercise.
- Differentiate between high impact and low impact aerobics.
- Describe step and slide aerobics.

KEY TERMS

While reading this chapter, you will become familiar with the following terms:

- ▶ Aerobics
- ▶ Aerobic Dance Exercise
- ▶ High Impact Aerobics

- ▶ Low Impact Aerobics
- ▶ Step Aerobics
- ▶ Slide Training

AEROBICS

What picture comes to mind when you hear the term *aerobics*? It may be a dance exercise class like the one you are about to begin. You may know that the term aerobic means with oxygen and became part of our exercise vocabulary in the late 1960s and early 1970s when Dr. Kenneth Cooper wrote his book Aerobics. Dr. Cooper's advice, at that time, was directed primarily to the American public to motivate them to begin some form of endurance exercise program as a preventative health measure to help reduce the risk of developing heart disease. Cooper's book emphasized participation in individual activities that require little or no equipment, such as cycling, jogging, swimming, and walking. Although many people did initiate a workout regimen, another form of exercise, known as aerobic dance, became a popular alternative when music was combined with vigorous dance. Jackie Sorenson and Judy Sheppard-Missett started the craze in the early 1970s by offering "jazzy" dance routines choreographed to popular music. Today, if there is an **aerobics** class going on, it's not running; it's some form of group exercise to music.

EVOLUTION OF AEROBIC DANCE EXERCISE

SAFETY AND EFFECTIVENESS

Aerobic dance exercise has changed significantly over the years. One improvement is increased safety and effectiveness of aerobics classes. Largely because of improved instructor training, certification, and research, aerobic dance has become a field in which exercise leaders have the opportunity to develop both technical and practical skills. A number of national and international organizations provide ongoing training and certification of instructors (see Appendix). In addition, most instructors rely on guidelines developed by The American College of Sports Medicine (ACSM) for program development and the ability to make recommendations for individual participants. The ACSM Position Stand on Developing and Maintaining Fitness in Healthy Adults is considered the "gold standard" in the fitness industry; it is used by most professionals because it is based on the best published research in the field of exercise science. Quality instruction requires a commitment to continuing education and constant analysis of movement selection and workout design. Excellent instructors make it seem easy to teach aerobics, but a great class reflects an ability to apply extensive knowledge of anatomy, physiology, and biomechanics—and make it fun!

CLASS VARIETY

Another change in the field of dance exercise is the wide variety of classes available today. Aerobic dance initially attracted mainly women, yet today's classes are more heterogeneous and most facilities offer numerous types of classes.

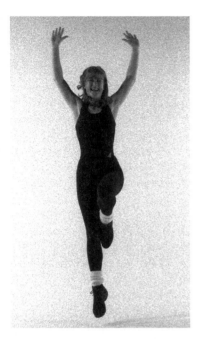

FIGURE 1-1 High impact aerobic movement (knee lift + hop).

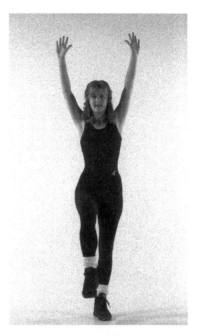

FIGURE 1-2 Low impact aerobic movement (knee lift + no hop).

Traditional aerobic dance exercise is vigorous, continuous movement performed to music and may be either high or low impact, or a combination of both.

A **high impact aerobics** class generally has bouncing or hopping movements and is most comparable to jogging in caloric expenditure and the force of impact (Figure 1-1). A **low impact aerobics** class eliminates the bouncing (Figure 1-2), and because one foot remains on the ground at all times, the impact of this exercise is similar to that of walking; however, its caloric expenditure can vary tremendously, depending on choreographic style and technique.

▶ **Aerobics**
Any activity requiring the presence of oxygen for the production of energy.

▶ **Aerobic Dance Exercise**
A popular alternative to traditional aerobic activities that combines music with vigorous dance-related movement.

▶ **High Impact Aerobics**
Aerobic activity that consists of bouncing or hopping movements and expends amounts of energy similar to those in jogging.

▶ **Low Impact Aerobics**
Aerobic activity that eliminates bouncing and jarring movements (one foot remains on the ground at all times), with greatly varying caloric expenditure because of the choreographic style and technique of the instructor.

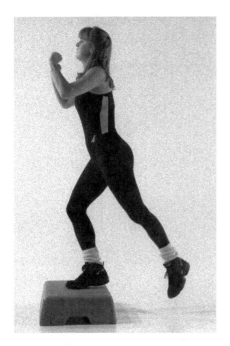

FIGURE 1-3 Step training.

Step training, or **step aerobics**, is another form of dance exercise, which became extremely popular with both men and women in the late 1980s. Using a stationary platform, participants perform a variety of stepping and upper body movement patterns to music. By varying the height of the step, each participant can personalize the workout to fit his or her own fitness level. Step training, which has relatively low impact forces, can range from a low to a high intensity workout, so that one instructor can accommodate a wide range of fitness levels in one class. Interestingly, step training seems to have attracted more men than other forms of dance exercise and may be more appealing because workouts often use resistive equipment and sport, rather than dance movement patterns (Figure 1-3).

Slide training uses mainly lateral movements, performed on a 4- to 6-foot commercially available slide (Figure 1-4). Because of the time required for equipment setup, safety concerns while the person is on or around the slide, and difficulty in learning or modifying the various sliding movements, slide training

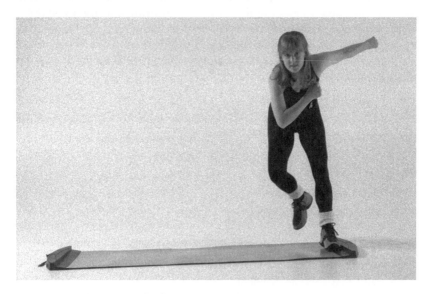

FIGURE 1-4 Slide training.

is usually a segment of a class. In other specialty classes, such as funk, hip-hop, and jazz, the instructor adapts a given form of dance for a group exercise setting.

SELECTING A PROGRAM THAT IS RIGHT FOR YOU

Is one of these forms of aerobic dance better for you than another? That depends! It depends on **you**: What are your goals and what are you trying to accomplish? The focus of this book is to help you look at the "big picture" and adopt aerobic dance as one part of a healthy lifestyle. We will examine the many positive effects of aerobic dance on body composition, aerobic fitness, muscular strength and endurance, and flexibility. We will also explore additional benefits from participating in regular aerobic exercise, such as increased energy and productivity. You will have the opportunity to establish personal goals in each of these areas, and—as you gain knowledge and expertise—to fine-tune those goals to help you maximize the benefits of this class. Finally, you will explore the wide world of exercise and see how it can fit into your lifestyle now and in the future. Get ready—for a lifetime of fitness!

SUMMARY

- The emphasis on aerobic exercise as a preventive health measure and the development of cardiorespiratory endurance began in the late 1960s and early 1970s.
- Aerobic dance exercise classes have changed over the years to improve safety and the effectiveness of the time spent in the activity.
- The American College of Sports Medicine and a number of other national and international organizations provide guidelines for training and are instrumental in the education of aerobic exercise instructors.
- As more people realize the health benefits of aerobic dance exercise, participants in aerobics classes are beginning to transcend sexual and age barriers.
- Analyzing your personal fitness goals and having the right information at hand will help you in deciding what type of aerobic dance exercise is right for you!

▶ **Step Aerobics**
Aerobic activity, first popular in the late 1980s, in which aerobic classes use a stationary platform and combine a variety of upper body movements. Intensity level can be modified to the person, and classes can accommodate persons with both low and high levels of fitness.

▶ **Slide Training**
Aerobic activity performed on a 4- to 6-foot slide; it is usually a segment of class because of safety concerns and the difficulty of learning or modifying the various slide movements.

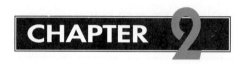

CHAPTER 2

UNDERSTANDING THE BIG PICTURE

OBJECTIVES

After reading this chapter, you should be able to do the following:

- Identify the four primary risk factors for the development of coronary artery disease.
- Describe the components of a well-rounded fitness program.
- Discuss the four basic training principles.

KEY TERMS

While reading this chapter, you will become familiar with the following terms:

- ► Body Composition
- ► Cardiorespiratory Endurance/Aerobic Fitness
- ► Components of Fitness
- ► Coronary Heart Disease
- ► Flexibility

Continued on p. 7.

KEY TERMS

Continued from p. 6.

- ► **Individual Differences**
- ► **Muscular Strength and Endurance**

- ► **Overload**
- ► **Reversibility**
- ► **Specificity**

THE FITNESS PUZZLE

Think of your life as being like a puzzle. When you look at the individual pieces, they don't have much meaning, but, when linked together, they form a beautiful picture. Aerobic dance exercise is one piece of the fitness puzzle, and fitness is one piece of a healthy lifestyle. Unlike a puzzle, though, your body has both an internal and an external component. Although right now you may be thinking only of working on the external, or how you *look*, one of the major benefits of exercise is how it affects the internal, or how you *function and feel*. Regular exercise can have a positive physical, mental, and emotional impact, because it affects your body in a number of ways as detailed in the accompanying box.

Internal and External Benefits of Regular Physical Activity

Internal

Physiologically:
- Improves the way your body functions and reduces certain health risks.
- Assists you in the performance of activities of daily living, recreation, and leisure.

Psychologically:
- Improves your self-esteem as a result of doing something good for yourself.
- Reduces stress.

External

Appearance: A fit and healthy appearance can increase confidence in how you present yourself socially and professionally.

THE DANGER OF INACTIVITY

The American Heart Association has identified four primary risk factors for the development of **coronary heart disease**: smoking, high blood pressure, high cholesterol levels, and physical inactivity. Physical inactivity is of tremendous concern because it affects so many more individuals than any of the other risk factors; in fact, more Americans are physically inactive than almost the total of the other three risk factors combined!

What are some of the benefits of regular exercise? They include the following:

- Reduced risk of developing coronary heart disease, osteoporosis or other lifestyle related diseases
- Reduced stress level
- Improved fitness level
- Improved recovery time
- Improved posture and body awareness
- Improved ability to perform daily functions

As you become more fit, you will probably notice that you have more energy and may be able to handle the challenges that come your way more easily, whether it is a written test or a workout. The increased self-confidence you develop by achieving your fitness goals may be the major reason you continue exercising long after you accomplish your physical goals.

COMPONENTS AND PRINCIPLES OF AN EXERCISE PROGRAM

Many persons begin an exercise program because they are interested in getting in shape, firming up, or reducing stress. Aerobic dance exercise is a great way to accomplish any of these goals, because it targets all of the **components of fitness: cardiorespiratory endurance/aerobic fitness, flexibility, muscular strength and endurance,** and **body composition.** Each of these components is a different piece of the puzzle that forms a well-rounded fitness program and will be discussed in detail later in this chapter.

FOUR BASIC TRAINING PRINCIPLES

Each aspect of fitness is developed and improved by applying four **basic training principles: overload, specificity, reversibility,** and **individual differences.** We will discuss these principles of training before looking at the components of fitness.

▶ Principle of Overload

Defined: Applying increased amounts of stress improves a targeted component of fitness.

Applied: Increasing the frequency, intensity or duration of an activity, or varying the type of exercise performed, improves a particular component of fitness.

You typically think of overload with strength training. Heavier weights with fewer repetitions are linked with greater strength gains, while lighter weights with more repetitions are associated with muscular endurance. Increasing the weight lifted is the best method for increasing strength, while increasing the number of

---

▶ **Coronary Heart Disease**

A major but often preventable disease that results from the accumulation of fatty deposits within the coronary arteries. Contributing factors are physical inactivity, smoking, high blood pressure, and high cholesterol.

▶ **Components of Fitness**

All well-rounded fitness programs should address cardiorespiratory endurance/aerobic fitness, flexibility, muscular strength and endurance, and body composition.

▶ **Cardiorespiratory Endurance/Aerobic Fitness**

The ability of the heart, lungs, and blood vessels to deliver oxygen and nutrients effectively and to remove waste products from working muscles over time.

▶ **Flexibility**

The ability to move through a full, normal range of motion and readily adapt to changes in position.

▶ **Muscular Strength**

The ability to exert a maximal force with a muscle or group of muscles.

▶ **Muscular Endurance**

The ability to contract a muscle or group of muscles repeatedly or to maintain continuous, low levels of muscular contraction.

▶ **Body Composition**

The types of tissues making up the body; they are divided into two components: lean weight (bones, organs, muscles) and fat weight.

▶ **Overload**

Application of increased amounts of stress to improve a targeted component of fitness.

▶ **Specificity**

The direct relationship between improvement or change and the type of overload applied.

▶ **Reversibility**

The "use it or lose it" principle. Your body will "detrain" by adapting to *not* exercising just as it trains by adapting to regular exercise.

▶ **Individual Differences**

The varying ways in which different persons respond to identical training programs.

repetitions is the best method to increase the overload to improve muscular endurance. As you increase strength, you need to lift heavier weights to continue to overload the muscle. The principle of overload also applies to the other components of fitness. If you want to promote flexibility of the hamstrings, vary the stretch or stretch more frequently. To overload the cardiovascular system, you could extend the aerobic segment of your workout or add another day or type of aerobic exercise each week.

Proper progression of overload enhances the effectiveness, safety, and enjoyment of exercise. Chapter 5 will help you develop realistic expectations for your exercise program, and subsequent chapters will address appropriate overload progressions for each of the components of fitness.

▶ Principle of Specificity

Defined: Improvement or change is directly related and restricted to the type of overload applied.

Applied: This principle is easy to see when comparing the components of fitness. For example, stretching will increase flexibility, but it will not make you stronger. Strengthening the calves does not affect your aerobic capacity. If you want to see change or improvement in a component of fitness, you need to train that component. If you want to gain strength, you must overload the muscular system. If you want to improve your aerobic fitness, overload the cardiovascular system with some form of aerobic activity. This principle also applies within each component of fitness. A training program that focuses on strengthening the upper body will not improve the strength of the lower body; the workouts would need to include exercises specific to the muscles of the lower body to see gains in that area. Similarly, stretching the calves will not improve the flexibility of the shoulder joint.

▶ Principle of Reversibility

Defined: This is also known as the "use it or lose it" principle. Your body will "detrain" by adapting to *not* exercising just as it trains by adapting to regular exercise.

Applied: Many students learn how to improve aerobic fitness, but they often wonder how quickly they will lose fitness if they stop exercising. Loss of cardiovascular endurance can be measured within 7 to 10 days of discontinuing exercise. You will return to pretraining levels (as if you had never exercised before) in 10 weeks to 8 months. The rate of detraining depends on factors such as genetics, your cardiovascular fitness level before stopping exercise, how long you had been fit before stopping, and your routine level of activity.

Cardiovascular fitness levels, however, can be maintained (not improved) with relatively little exercise. Some research has shown that you can reduce training frequency and duration by up to two thirds and still maintain cardiovascular fitness levels for up to 15 weeks *if* you maintain your training intensity. This means that, for example, if you currently work out 3 days a week for 60 minutes at a "somewhat hard" pace, you would stay at your same level of fitness for a period of time with only one 60-minute workout a week *if* you kept the intensity at somewhat hard.

How can you use this information? If you are swamped with exams, work, travel or other obligations, get at least one good workout in each week and return to your normal training schedule as soon as possible. There are similar findings in the research concerning muscular strength and endurance.

▶ Principle of Individual Differences

Defined: Different persons will respond to identical training programs in a slightly different fashion.

Applied: In simple terms, do not compare yourself to anyone else. If someone in your class started the semester at exactly the same level of fitness as you (not very likely!), you would both improve, but not in exactly the same way or by the same amount. Improvement in each of the components of fitness is affected by your current level of fitness, your training program, your general lifestyle, and your genetics. More and more research is demonstrating that your genetics play an important role in how you respond to exercise. One participant might, for example, see dramatic body composition changes, while another who worked just as hard might see very little change. A more muscular person may respond to resistance training more quickly than a tall, thin person. This information is not to discourage you from working hard, only to discourage you from comparing yourself to anyone else. There is only one you, and you will respond to exercise in a unique way. You have not been manufactured like a common puzzle picture; *You* are an original! The key is to find a workout plan that works for you and stick with it.

COMPONENTS OF FITNESS

▶ Cardiorespiratory Endurance or Aerobic Fitness

Defined: This is the ability of the heart, lungs, and blood vessels to deliver oxygen and nutrients effectively and to remove waste products from working muscles over time.

Applied: Generally regarded as the most important component of physical fitness, cardiovascular endurance is also referred to as *aerobic fitness, cardiopulmonary fitness, cardiorespiratory endurance,* and a variety of other terms referring to the efficiency of the heart and lungs to deliver and use oxygen. For simplicity's sake, we will use *aerobic fitness* for the remainder of this book. The best measure of aerobic fitness is maximal oxygen uptake: the amount of oxygen a person is capable of utilizing per minute when working at 100%. Your aerobic capacity is best improved through activities that demand increasing amounts of oxygen and challenge the ability of the heart to pump blood and deliver oxygen for the muscles to use. These aerobic activities rely predominately on moving the large muscles of the lower body repetitively over extended periods of time and requiring the body to take in and utilize large quantities of oxygen. A few examples of popular activities that are aerobic include running, cycling, swimming, walking, dance exercise, and rowing.

To improve the condition of the cardiovascular system, you must overload the system, or ask it to do more than it is used to doing by manipulating the frequency, intensity, or duration of your aerobic activity. For instance, if you are used to walking for exercise and you decide to jog, you've increased the intensity of the workout to provide an overload for the cardiovascular system. You could also have increased the number of days you walk each week or increased the number of minutes you walk. See the Fitness Tip on this page for more information.

What should you do to make sure your workout is "aerobic?" The American College of Sports Medicine (ACSM) has established guidelines for improving or maintaining aerobic fitness based on the most comprehensive research in the field of exercise science. The ACSM recommends that you exercise *3 to 5 days a week*, for a duration of *20 to 60 minutes*, at an intensity you would describe as *somewhat hard* to *hard*. Understanding how to exercise within these ranges will help you design a workout program that meets your goals and schedule. These variables will be discussed in depth in Chapter 8.

▶ Flexibility

Defined: Flexibility is the ability to move through a full, normal range of motion and readily adapt to changes in position.

Applied: There are two main types of flexibility: static and dynamic. Static flexibility is the ability to assume a particular position with no regard to speed. Dynamic flexibility is the ability to move through the full range of motion at normal or higher speeds of movement, such as a split leap or high kick.

Fitness Tip

Developing Cardiovascular Endurance

Overload: Work harder, longer, more frequently. Example: Begin with a 20-minute aerobic segment you would classify as *somewhat hard*; progress to a 30-minute aerobic segment you would describe as *hard*.

Specificity: Aerobic work will improve the cardiovascular system. The best way to improve performance of a particular activity is to train that way. If performance is not the goal, most activities will have similar training effects if you expend the same total number of calories.

Reversibility: You will lose fitness gains if you completely stop training; maintain fitness with fewer workouts of the same intensity.

Individual differences: Your aerobic capacity has a genetic maximum; you will see the greatest fitness gains at the start of a program.

Static flexibility is particularly important in being able to maintain good alignment when you are sitting or standing still. Tight muscles pull the body out of alignment, causing muscular imbalance and uneven wear and tear on the joints. Dynamic flexibility is the ability to move through a range of motion at normal or higher speeds. This is the type of flexibility required for sports and vigorous activities. It is active flexibility and includes an element of strength and coordinated action among muscle groups.

Flexibility is joint-specific. That is, a person might have tightness at the ankles but be very flexible at the shoulders. Flexibility may also differ from right to left sides. Flexibility can be measured by degrees of movement, but is usually defined simply as normal, limited, or excessive.

To improve in flexibility you must stretch every day. Some experts say twice a day, particularly if you are training for a sport like gymnastics. There will be little if any progress with less frequent stretching.

To improve static flexibility you must overload the muscular system with regard to length. This is called applying an overstretch. Overstretch is the point at the end of the current range of motion where a sensation of stretch is felt but does not result in pain. Pain can cause a reflexive rebound effect of increased tightness. Static stretches should be held for 30 to 60 seconds. Taking long, deep breaths while holding a stretch promotes relaxation and decreases muscle tension. Three to five breaths is a convenient way to time a static stretch.

To improve dynamic flexibility, you must take another step, from passive to active stretch, from holding to moving through the range of motion. Move through the available range of motion at normal speeds or at the velocities required for a particular activity. See the Fitness Tip below for more information.

Fitness Tip

Improving Flexibility

Overload: Stretch farther, differently, or longer. Example: Start with a standing "wall" calf stretch; progress to a standing "stair" calf stretch.

Specificity: Stretch muscles that are tight; strengthen those that are weak.

Reversibility: Loss of flexibility will occur without continued stretching, particularly in the muscles of the hips and upper torso because of habitual postures in daily living.

Individual differences: You may have very flexible hips because of your genetic make-up, requiring minimal stretching; someone else may need to stretch repeatedly throughout the day to achieve normal flexibility of the hip joints.

▶ Muscular Endurance

Defined: Muscular endurance is the ability to contract a muscle or group of muscles repeatedly or to maintain continuous, low levels of muscular contraction.

Applied: Improvement of muscular endurance will lead to an increased ability to perform sustained muscular contractions, whether in routine daily activities such as walking, or specific to a particular sport, such as cycling. The best way to improve muscular endurance is to perform an action repeatedly with an amount of resistance that allows you to complete about 20 repetitions. Muscular endurance is related to your level of muscular strength: you must be strong enough to perform a particular motion. By repeating the action many times, you are also working on muscular endurance. Whether you work primarily on strength or endurance depends on the amount of weight lifted and the number of repetitions completed. Muscular endurance is best developed by lifting a relatively low amount of weight many times. The Fitness Tip below provides additional information on improving your muscular endurance.

▶ Muscular Strength

Defined: The ability to exert a maximal force with a muscle or group of muscles is muscular strength.

Applied: Because strength measures the amount of weight you can lift just one time, muscular strength is not typically a focus in aerobic programs. Increasing muscular strength requires **overloading** the muscular system by using increasing

Fitness Tip

Enhancing Muscular Endurance

Overload: Perform muscular contractions repeatedly to the point of fatigue or muscular failure. For example, start with 10 push-ups without stopping; build to 50 push-ups.

Specificity: Repetitive movements improve the ability of a muscle to continue to perform that activity; they do not lead to spot reduction or to burning fat from a particular area of the body.

Reversibility: Without continued training, muscles are not able to sustain repeated contractions.

Individual differences: You may have a higher capacity for muscular endurance exercises because of your particular muscle-fiber type and body structure.

amounts of resistance. Muscular strength is best improved by lifting the amount of weight that causes your muscles to completely fatigue after 8 to 12 repetitions: you should be physically unable to perform repetition number 13. The ACSM states that measurable strength gains can be achieved by performing *one set of 8 to 12 repetitions at least 2 days a week for the major muscle groups.* Increasing the number of sets and repetitions does not lead to significantly greater strength gains. Those seeking significant muscle hypertrophy for competitive reasons often use multiple sets of exercises. However, research demonstrates that one set, properly overloaded, gives excellent increases in strength. The Fitness Tip below summarizes a sound approach for increasing muscular strength.

▶ Body Composition

Defined: Your total body weight is divided into two components: lean weight (bones, organs, muscles) and fat weight. Your weight as measured on a scale represents your total body weight and is the combination of these two weights.

Applied: Evaluating body composition is the best means of knowing what you should weigh, because body composition makes the distinction between *fat* and *weight*. General recommendations are that men and women should be 15% to 20% and 20% to 26% body fat, respectively. Competitive athletes are often significantly leaner than these values.

Fitness Tip

Increasing Muscular Strength

Overload: Perform muscular contractions against increasing amounts of external resistance. Example: Start with a bench press weight of 40 pounds for 8 repetitions; progress to 10 repetitions, then 12 repetitions. Increase to 50 pounds for 8, then 10, then 12 repetitions.

Specificity: Resistance training will improve muscular strength; despite high heart rates, it is not an aerobic activity.

Reversibility: Without continued overload, strength gains will plateau; loss of muscle mass can occur in untrained body parts without ongoing training.

Individual differences: How your body responds to strength training reflects your genetics and the intensity of your training. With similar training programs, some women can significantly improve strength without changing muscle size, while others will see measurable increase in muscle size.

The best way to lose fat weight and maintain muscle mass is by combining aerobic exercise with a healthy, low-calorie eating plan (see Fitness Tip below). Aerobic exercise will increase total caloric expenditure and possibly increase lean tissue slightly. Resistance training, particularly with heavier weights, is the most effective means of increasing muscle mass. Reducing the number of total calories and fat calories consumed will reduce your amount of excess body fat. Increasing muscle while losing fat will enable you to work more efficiently with less risk of injury, and you will look better, feel lighter, and have more energy.

By keeping your focus on fitness and body composition as part of the big picture, you can learn to recognize the internal as well as the external progress you are making. Do not get hung up on weighing in to evaluate your program: look instead at how your clothes fit and think about how you feel, and you'll get a more valid picture than your scale weight can give you!

SUMMARY

- Increasing your level of aerobic fitness has a number of benefits, including an improved level of overall fitness, enhancing your self image, and decreasing your risk of coronary artery disease.
- Aerobic dance exercise targets the necessary components of any fitness program: aerobic endurance, flexibility, muscular strength and endurance, and body composition.
- Keeping in mind the training principles of overload, specificity, reversibility, and individual differences will assist you in meeting your fitness goals and increase your chances of sticking to your program.

Fitness Tip

Reducing Body Fat

Lean weight vs fat weight:

- Increase your weekly time spent exercising to 3 to 5 days a week for 20 to 60 minutes at time.
- Decrease fat and total caloric intake by eating a healthy, well-balanced diet.

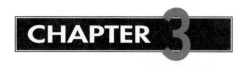

CHAPTER 3

BASIC FITNESS ASSESSMENTS

OBJECTIVES

After reading this chapter, you should be able to do the following:

- Explain the difference between maximal and submaximal fitness tests.
- Accurately and consistently monitor your heart rate.
- Apply fitness assessments that measure your current level of health, aerobic fitness, flexibility, and muscular strength and endurance.
- Evaluate your fitness assessments to help you *plan, prioritize,* and *modify* your workout to achieve realistic goals for both the short and long term.

KEY TERMS

While reading this chapter, you will become familiar with the following terms:

- ▶ Basal Metabolic Rate
- ▶ Body Mass Index
- ▶ Energy Balance
- ▶ Girth Measurement
- ▶ Health Risk Appraisal
- ▶ Submaximal Tests
- ▶ Vo_2max

BEFORE YOU SET YOUR FITNESS GOALS

To set your fitness goals, it is important to assess your fitness levels before you begin your program. Results from the assessments form the baseline for comparison by which you can measure your progress and see the results of your efforts at the end of the term. The assessments will include Health Risk Appraisal and measurements of aerobic fitness, body mass index, girths, basal metabolic rate, posture, flexibility, and muscular strength and endurance.

The results of these assessments will help you *plan, prioritize,* and *modify* your workouts. For example, if you see that you are very flexible at the shoulders but have tight hip muscles, plan to stretch your hips and thighs more frequently than your shoulders. If your aerobic fitness is good but your flexibility is poor, make stretching a priority until you are more balanced and less likely to be injured. Tight hip muscles may also require you to modify certain abdominal, back, or hip exercises to accommodate your tightness until you gain the needed flexibility in that area.

HEALTH RISK APPRAISAL

The first element of fitness assessment is a **health risk appraisal** (HRA), found in Assessment 3-1. The purpose of the HRA is to look at your health history and current lifestyle as well as to identify any special physical conditions or medications that may require specific exercise modifications. Part A, the Physical Activity Readiness Questionnaire (PAR-Q) will help you determine if you should seek medical advice before beginning an exercise program. Part B, the HRA itself, evaluates your physical activity level, lifestyle, and eating behaviors.

Another important area of assessment is your intake of dietary fat. To supplement the information gained from the HRA, use Assessment 3-2, created by Consumer Reports to gauge your dietary fat intake.

PREDICTING YOUR RESTING METABOLIC RATE

To maintain your body weight, you need to be in what is called energy balance. This means that the number of calories you take in (through eating and drinking) is equal to the number of calories you expend (through activity and other metabolic processes). Theoretically, if you can unbalance this equation, you should be able to gain or lose weight. If you take in more calories than you expend you will gain weight; if you take in fewer calories than you expend you should lose weight. This formula is a good rule of thumb, but it does not always work because there are so many factors that can affect your metabolism.

Your **resting metabolic rate** (RMR), also known as basal metabolic rate (BMR), is the minimum amount of energy your body requires to function at complete rest. Your RMR accounts for about 60% to 75% of your total energy expenditure in a day. Other factors include the thermic effect of a meal (TEM), which is the increase in metabolism seen after eating, and the thermic effect of activity (TEA). TEM accounts for about 10% and TEA 15% to 30% of your total energy expenditure.

Most of the variability in RMR seems to be caused by age, sex, and lean body mass. In general, RMR is higher in males than females, in younger adults than older adults, and in heavier rather than lighter persons. Assessment 3-3 will help you predict your RMR to give you an idea of how many calories your body needs to function each day; any activity you perform will require additional energy. If you know about how many calories you burn during your exercise class, add that plus about 300 additional Calories for normal daily living to your predicted RMR to get an idea of about how many calories you need to consume each day to maintain your body weight. If you want to unbalance your energy equation for weight loss or gain, be sure that any increase or reduction in calories is minimal (about 300 to 500 Calories) and alter your activity levels accordingly.

AEROBIC FITNESS

A test for aerobic fitness is designed to measure your body's ability to use oxygen and sustain aerobic activity. During aerobic activity the muscles need oxygen to continue working, so they draw more oxygen out of the bloodstream. As the muscles demand more oxygen, more fresh blood must reach the muscle cells; therefore the blood vessels must dilate, the heart must beat faster and stronger, and the lungs must exchange air faster.

As you participate in aerobic training activities, each component of the oxygen use and delivery system will improve. The accompanying box on the following page summarizes the benefits of aerobic training.

There are several methods to measure aerobic fitness. The more sophisticated maximal graded exercise test, or stress test, directly measures your maximal oxygen uptake (Vo_2max). Your **Vo_2max** indicates how much oxygen your body can use when you are working as hard as you possibly can—your maximal capacity. The more oxygen you can consume, the better your aerobic condition.

▶ **Health Risk Appraisal**
A process of looking at one's health history and current lifestyle to identify conditions that may require specific exercise modifications.

▶ **Energy Balance**
A state in which the number of Calories you take in (through eating and drinking) is equal to the number of Calories you expend (through activity and other metabolic processes).

▶ **Resting (Basal) Metabolic Rate**
The minimum amount of energy your body requires to function at rest.

▶ **Vo_2max**
Maximal ability to uptake and use oxygen.

Benefits of Aerobic Training on Your Oxygen Use and Delivery System

You will see improvement through:
1. Increased ability of the muscle cells to use oxygen and burn fuel
2. Improved efficiency of the heart and vessels of the cardiovascular system to deliver and return blood
3. More efficient exchange of oxygen and carbon dioxide in the lungs

Most tests used in fitness centers are **submaximal tests**. They are designed to indirectly measure your body's ability to use oxygen by predicting your maximal capacity based on your heart rate during exercise. Submaximal tests are reasonably accurate and are much easier to administer than maximal stress tests. They provide a valuable way to measure improvement by comparing results before and after an exercise program.

The aerobic fitness test presented in Assessment 3-4 is a 3-minute step test. It measures your heart rate as you recover from a short bout of continuous exercise at a specific rate of speed. You will establish an initial fitness category based on the outcome of your step test. The results are based on research showing that a well-conditioned cardiovascular system will recover more quickly than an untrained one from an equal bout of exercise. If your aerobic fitness level improves over the course of this semester, you can expect your heart rate to be lower when you take the step test again, because your heart will be stronger and able to pump more blood with each beat. This means that your heart does not have to work as hard during the step test and is a good indicator that you are in r aerobic shape.

Several factors can affect the outcome of an indirect test like the step test. These variables include smoking, coffee consumption, certain medications, room temperature, fatigue, prior exercise, or simply miscounting the recovery heart rate. Be sure you are well-rested before taking a step test. Refrain from exercise, smoking, and drinking coffee before the test.

LEARNING TO TAKE YOUR PULSE

Accurate results of a step test depend on your ability to take your heart rate accurately. Your pulse can be measured at one of several sites by applying light pressure with the index and middle fingers. Do not use the thumb. A radial pulse is taken on the underside of the wrist on the same side as the thumb (Figure 3-1). A carotid pulse is measured just to the side of the windpipe (Figure 3-2).

It is important to begin counting the pulse within 5 seconds of stopping exercise. Begin counting the first beat as zero and the second beat as one in order not

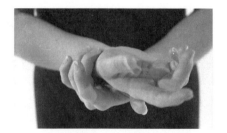

FIGURE 3-1 Radial pulse.

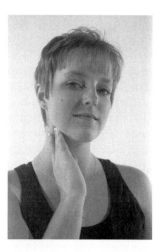

to overestimate the heart rate. Walk in place or step side to side while counting, because standing still immediately after vigorous activity may cause dizziness as a result of blood collecting in the lower part of the body.

FIGURE 3-2 Carotid pulse.

BODY MASS INDEX AND GIRTH MEASUREMENTS

More important than knowing your height and weight is knowing your percentage of body fat. When you are seeking to lose weight, you need to set goals in terms of losing fat, not just weight. Body composition testing identifies what percentage of your body weight is lean weight (bones, organs, muscles) and what percentage is fat weight. The most accurate method of testing is underwater or hydrostatic weighing. Other methods include bioelectrical impedance and skinfolds. Check with your instructor because these tests may be available at a university, medical center, or fitness facility.

One measure of your body weight that has some value, however, is your **body mass index** (BMI). Your BMI is related to body composition because it is correlated to percent of body fat. BMI is the standard many insurance and government agencies use to determine whether you are "officially" overweight. Researchers determine BMI by dividing body weight in kilograms by the square of body height in meters. You can use Assessment 3-5 to calculate your BMI. A BMI of 27.8 or higher for men or 27.3 or higher for women is considered too high and would indicate that you are at risk of health problems related to body weight.

▶ **Submaximal Tests**
Based on measurements of heart rate during exercise, these tests are fairly accurate at predicting one's maximal oxygen capacity.

▶ **Body Mass Index**
A ratio of body weight to height that is used by insurance and government agencies to determine whether a person is "officially" overweight.

GIRTH MEASUREMENTS

Another method to measure change in body size is to take simple **girth measurements** (Figure 3-3). By measuring different body parts you will be able to determine whether you are changing size, which can be an indicator of changing body composition. Working with a partner, use a measuring tape at the body parts listed in Assessment 3-6 and record the measurements. Be sure to measure each body part at the largest circumference (widest) or smallest circumference (narrowest) as indicated. While you complete the assessment, it is important to note whether you measure on the right or left side of the body. If possible, measure directly on the skin, since clothing will affect your values. Because a change of even ¼ inch is significant, measure as carefully as possible. Try to have the same partner repeat the measurements at the end of the semester.

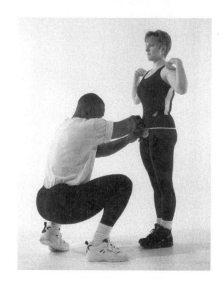

FIGURE 3-3 Girth Measurements.

FLEXIBILITY TESTING

Your range of movement at a particular joint is known as your flexibility. The amount of movement that is possible for you at each joint is determined by the structure and alignment of the bones forming the joint, the tightness of the joint capsule enclosing the joint, and the stiffness of the ligaments, tendons, and muscles surrounding the joint. In some cases, excess fat or muscle (in body-builders) may limit the amount of movement that can occur at a specific joint.

Flexibility is specific for each joint. For example, you may be very flexible at your shoulders but have tight hip joints. Flexibility can also differ from side to side. Your left knee may show normal flexibility, while your right knee is tight.

Your flexibility is also influenced by your age, gender, and level of activity. Younger people are usually more flexible than older people because aging (and inactivity) causes the connective tissues to become less elastic. Active people are sometimes more flexible than inactive people because inactivity causes stiffness of the muscles, connective tissue, and joints. However, athletes sometimes become selectively tight in certain areas because of the repetitive nature of practicing and playing a specific sport. These selective areas of inflexibility and muscle imbalance are often the cause of sports injuries. For example, runners often have very tight hip joints. Some people are genetically more flexible than others, no matter what they do.

Hips, shoulders, knees, and ankles are the joints most frequently affected by reduced flexibility. Many people are tight or inflexible because of habitual postures—positions in which they hold their bodies for much of the day. Because many people sit much of the day, the hips and knees are flexed for long periods of time. Sitting with crossed legs can produce even more tightness on one side. The chest is often collapsed forward with the spine flexed forward. The shoulders are held close to the body and rolled inward and forward.

When muscles are held in a shortened position and are never stretched, they adapt to the position by becoming even shorter and tighter. Also with inactivity, tissues become stiff and more difficult to move. Therefore if you sit much of the day without stretching and without vigorous activity, the muscles of the hips knees, ankles, shoulders and torso can become stiff and tight over time. Static stretching in the opposite direction can prevent muscle shortening. For example, if your shoulders roll forward most of the day, take time to rotate them back and press them down periodically throughout the day. If your hips and knees are always flexed, periodically stretch them into extension.

Inflexible joints and muscles can also cause excess fatigue and uneven wear-and tear on the joints. For example, tightness of the structures on the outside of the knee can pull the kneecap too far to the outside, causing the underside to scrape against the femur, especially as you bend and straighten the knee and as you climb stairs, lunge forward on a bent knee, or bend down to lift something from the floor. This can lead to damage of the cartilage behind the kneecap.

Joints are designed to move within a specific range of motion. Too much flexibility can be just as much a problem as a lack of flexibility. Many dancers and gymnasts strive to become hyperflexible, but they may pay a price for it later with unstable joints. The middle back may be overstretched in students who sit all day with their shoulders rounded forward to read or work at a desk. This overstretched condition can also lead to shoulder problems, headaches, even neck or wrist problems.

Testing your flexibility is important in tailoring a workout to meet your individual needs. Spend extra time outside class, stretching the areas that appear to be overly tight. The box on the next page lists guidelines for performing the flexibility tests in Assessments 3-7 to 3-10 at the end of this chapter.

▶ **Girth Measurements**

Measurements of different body parts (biceps, chest, waist, hips, thigh, and calf) that, repeated consistently over a period of time, can be an indicator of changing body composition.

Guidelines for Flexibility Assessment

1. Dress in nonbinding exercise clothing that allows freedom of movement and visual assessment of joint angles. A leotard and tights or shorts and a T-shirt are appropriate.
2. Assume the "start" position as illustrated.
3. Perform the indicated action for the specific joint or muscle.
4. Hold at the end of the range of motion, where you feel tension in the muscle or tendon. Do not press to the point of pain.
5. Do not try to look flexible by twisting or overstretching another body part. Get the real picture of where you are, so real improvements can occur.
6. Do not force a position, bounce, or continue with a position that causes discomfort.
7. Have your partner compare your final position to the illustrations of normal, limited, or excessive range of motion.
8. Record your results after each test. Scores should reflect a normal (N), limited (L), or excessive (E) range as pictured.

At the end of this chapter are additional worksheets designed to help you complete the information on your fitness assessment. Assessment 3-11 is a muscular strength and endurance push-up test. Assessment 3-12 is an abdominal stabilization test (leg lowering test), and Assessment 3-13 is a comprehensive postural assessment.

SUMMARY

- Results from the fitness assessments in this chapter will form the baseline for comparison by which you can measure your progress and see the results of your efforts.
- To maintain a consistent body weight you need to maintain an energy balance. To lose weight you need to offset this balance by increasing your level of physical activity and/or decreasing your caloric intake by 300 to 500 Calories a day.
- Aerobic training has been shown to enhance the functioning of your oxygen use and delivery systems by increasing the efficiency of your muscle cells to burn oxygen, improving the efficiency of the circulatory system, and making the oxygen and carbon dioxide exchange in the lungs more efficient.
- Flexibility is influenced by age, gender, and level of activity. Testing your flexibility is an important part of tailoring a workout to meet your individual needs.

- Muscle strength and endurance are a continuum of well-developed muscle action and coordination. Strength and endurance assessment is also an important part of customizing your workout.
- Examining your posture is an important overview and summary of your musculoskeletal fitness. It demonstrates how well your strength and flexibility are integrated, producing a well-aligned and balanced body that can participate in aerobic and sports activities without injury.

Assessment 3-1

(A Questionnaire for People Aged 15 to 69)

Name	Section	Date

Regular physical activity is fun and healthy, and increasingly more people are starting to become more active every day. Being more active is very safe for most people. However, some people should check with their doctor before they start becoming much more physically active.

If you are planning to become much more physically active than you are now, start by answering the seven questions in the box below. If you are between the ages of 15 and 69, the PAR-Q will tell you if you should check with your doctor before you start. If you are over 69 years of age and you are not used to being very active, check with your doctor.

Common sense is your best guide when you answer these questions. Please read the questions carefully and answer each one honestly: check YES or NO. AFTER YOU HAVE DONE SO, GO ON TO THE NEXT PAGE.

YES NO

☐ ☐ 1. Has your doctor ever said that you have a heart condition *and* that you should only do physical activity recommended by a doctor?

☐ ☐ 2. Do you feel pain in your chest when you do physical activity?

☐ ☐ 3. In the past month, have you had chest pain when you were not doing physical activity?

☐ ☐ 4. Do you lose your balance because of dizziness or do you ever lose consciousness?

☐ ☐ 5. Do you have a bone or joint problem that could be made worse by a change in your physical activity?

☐ ☐ 6. Is your doctor currently prescribing drugs (for example, water pills) for your blood pressure or heart condition?

☐ ☐ 7. Do you know of *any other reason* why you should not do physical activity?

Continued on p. 28

27

YES to one or more questions

If

you

answered

Talk with your doctor by phone or in person *before* you start becoming much more physically active or *before* you have a fitness appraisal. Tell your doctor about the PAR-Q and which questions you answered YES.

- You may be able to do any activity you want—as long as you start slowly and build up gradually. Or, you may need to restrict your activities to those that are safe for you. Talk with your doctor about the kinds of activities you wish to participate in and follow his/her advice.
- Find out which community programs are safe and helpful for you.

NO to all questions

If you answered NO honestly to *all* PAR-Q questions, you can be reasonably sure that you can:

- Start becoming much more physically active—begin slowly and build up gradually. This is the safest and easiest way to go.
- Take part in a fitness appraisal—this is an excellent way to determine your basic fitness so that you can plan the best way for you to live actively.

DELAY BECOMING MUCH MORE ACTIVE:

- If you are not feeling well because of a temporary illness such as a cold or a fever—wait until you feel better; or
- If you are or may be pregnant—talk to your doctor before you start becoming more active.

Please note: if your health changes so that you then answer yes to any of the above questions, tell your fitness or health professional. Ask whether you should change your physical activity plan.

Informed use of the PAR-Q: The Canadian Society for Exercise Physiology, Health Canada, and their agents assume no liability for persons who undertake physical activity, and if in doubt after completing this questionnaire, consult your doctor before physical activity.

You are encouraged to copy the PAR-Q but only if you use the entire form.

NOTE: *If the PAR-Q is being given to a person before he or she participates in a physical activity program or a fitness appraisal, this section may be used for legal or administrative purposes.*

I have read, understood and completed this questionnaire. Any questions I had were answered to my full satisfaction.

Name_____

Signature _____

Signature of parent _____

or guardian (for participants under the age of majority)

Date _____ Witness_____

© Canadian Society for Exercise Physiology
Société canadienne de physiologie de l'exercice
Supported by: Health Canada   Santé Canada

Thomas S, Reading J, and Shephard RJ: Revision of the Physical Activity Readiness Questionnaire (PAR-Q). Can J Sport Sci 17:338-345, 1992 (based on the British Columbia Department of Health, PAR-Q Validation Report, 1975).

Part B. Health Risk Appraisal

PHYSICAL ACTIVITY LEVEL

How many days per week do you:
1. Engage in light to moderate physical activity (similar to sustained walking) at least 30 minutes/day?
   Never _____ 1-2 _____ 3-4 _____ >5 _____
2. Engage in vigorous physical activity 3 or more days/week for at least 20 minutes?
   Never _____ 1 _____ 2 _____ >3 _____
3. Perform some form of resistance training?
   Never _____ 1 _____ 2 _____ >3 _____

Comments for Physical Activity Questions 1-3: Although many experts are now recommending "light" levels of physical activity to improve health, more vigorous exercise is necessary to promote changes in fitness. If you do not exercise regularly, consider increasing your everyday physical activity (such as walking to class, taking the stairs rather than the elevator, etc.) to improve your health status. Adding in vigorous workouts combined with some resistance training should improve your fitness and health condition.

LIFESTYLE

Do you:
4. Use seat belts when driving/riding in motor vehicles?
   Never _____ Sometimes _____ Usually _____ Always _____
5. Limit exposure to the sun and use sunscreen and/or protective clothing when necessary?
   Never _____ Sometimes _____ Usually _____ Always _____
6. Experience significant stress?
   Never _____ Sometimes _____ Usually _____ Always _____
7. Take steps to control stresses in your life?
   Never _____ Sometimes _____ Usually _____ Always _____
8. Smoke?
   Yes _____ Ex-smoker _____ Never _____
9. Drink alcohol?
   Yes _____ No _____

Comments for Lifestyle Questions 4-9: Each of these areas identifies situations or conditions over which you have some control. Begin to recognize that you make daily choices that affect your overall well-being. Chronically high levels of stress, for instance, can be just as deadly as not wearing your seat belt. Consider making some positive lifestyle choices if you answered "yes" to any of these questions.

DIETARY ANALYSIS

Do you:

10. Eat 6 or more servings of grain products daily? (One serving = 1 slice of bread; ½ cup cooked cereal, rice or pasta; ½ bagel, muffin or bun; 1 small tortilla; 1 ounce of ready to eat cereal; etc.)

    Never _____ Sometimes _____ Usually _____ Always _____ Not sure _____

11. Eat 5 or more servings of fruits, vegetables, and legumes daily?

    Never _____ Sometimes _____ Usually _____ Always _____ Not sure _____

12. Eat 2 or more servings of calcium rich foods daily (dairy products, etc.)?

    Never _____ Sometimes _____ Usually _____ Always _____ Not sure _____

13. Keep dietary fat intake to 30% or less of your total calories?

    Never _____ Sometimes _____ Usually _____ Always _____ Not sure _____

14. Keep saturated fat intake to 10% or less of total calories?

    Never _____ Sometimes _____ Usually _____ Always _____ Not sure _____

Comments for Dietary Analysis Questions 10-14: It is helpful to look at the amount and type of foods you eat. If you were "not sure" about any of the answers above, you will find additional nutritional information in Chapters 6 and 7 to help you better understand and evaluate what you eat. Exercise is most effective when combined with a balanced, nutrient-dense diet that is adequate in calories, and low in fat and simple sugars. Increasing your intake of fruits, grains, and vegetables can affect your overall health by providing more energy and even reducing your risk of developing certain cancers. Adequate levels of dietary calcium are of particular importance for women who are at greater risk of developing osteoporosis, or bone loss. The main reason persons tend to be overfat, however, is too much fat in the diet. Often, fat is "hidden" in processed or prepared foods and it can be difficult to be certain how much fat you are consuming. If you are unsure about the amount of fat in your diet, use the following questionnaire. Check with your instructor or other nutrition professional if you are interested in a more thorough dietary analysis.

Assessment 3-2

Name   Section   Date

How well are you keeping extra fat out of your diet? One way to check is to keep a careful daily record of how many calories and grams of fat you eat. A much simpler way to check your fat consumption is to complete this new quiz, designed by researchers at Seattle's Fred Hutchinson Cancer Research Center, whose studies have found it a fairly accurate way to estimate consumption. The questionnaire also lets you know how well you're doing on five basic fat-cutting strategies recommended by dietitians. Think about your diet over the past three months and answer each of the following questions with a number from this list. If a question does not apply to your diet, leave it blank. (For instance, if you do not eat red meat, do not answer questions 5, 6, and 19—your score is based on the rest of your diet.)

1 = Usually/Always   3 = Sometimes
2 = Often   4 = Rarely/Never

QUIZ

In the past three months, when you—
1. Ate fish, did you avoid frying it? _____
2. Ate chicken, did you avoid frying it? _____
3. Ate chicken, did you remove the skin? _____
4. Ate spaghetti or noodles, did you eat it plain or with a meatless tomato sauce? _____
5. Ate red meat, did you trim all the visible fat? _____
6. Ate ground beef, did you choose extra lean? _____
7. Ate bread, rolls, or muffins, did you eat them without butter or margarine? _____
8. Drank milk, was it skim or 1% milk instead of 2% or whole? _____
9. Ate cheese, was it a reduced-fat variety? _____
10. Ate a frozen dessert, was it sherbet, ice milk, or nonfat yogurt or ice cream? _____
11. Ate cooked vegetables, did you eat them *without* adding butter, margarine, salt pork, or bacon fat? _____
12. Ate cooked vegetables, did you avoid frying them? _____
13. Ate potatoes, were they cooked by a method other than frying? _____
14. Ate boiled or baked potatoes, did you eat them *without* butter, margarine, or sour cream? _____

15. Ate green salads with dressing, did you use a low-fat or nonfat dressing? _____
16. Ate dessert, did you eat only fruit? _____
17. Ate a snack was it raw vegetables? _____
18. Ate a snack, was it fresh fruit? _____
19. Cooked red meat, did you trim all the fat before cooking? _____
20. Used mayonnaise or a mayonnaise-type dressing, was it low-fat or nonfat? _____

SCORING

To estimate the percentage of Calories from fat in your diet, transfer the numbers above to the score sheet below. Disregard questions that were left blank. (Note that the items are arranged within five fat-lowering strategies rather than according to their order in the quiz.) Figure your average score for each of the strategies (the total divided by the number of answers you gave). Add up the five averages and divide by five. Then check the chart.

Strategy 1: Avoid frying	Strategy 3: Avoid fat as flavoring	Strategy 5: Replace fatty foods with produce
Items:	Items:	Items:
1 _____	4 _____	16 _____
2 _____	7 _____	17 _____
12 _____	11 _____	18 _____
13 _____	14 _____	
Subtotal _____	Subtotal _____	Subtotal _____
Average _____	Average _____	Average _____
Strategy 2: Modify meat	Strategy 4: Substitute low-fat or nonfat versions	Overall score _____ (sum of 5 averages):
Items:	Items:	
3 _____	8 _____	Divide overall score
5 _____	9 _____	by 5 to get overall
6 _____	10 _____	average:
19 _____	15 _____	
Subtotal _____	20 _____	_____
Average _____	Subtotal _____	
	Average _____	

If overall average is. . .		Your % of fats from Calories is. . .	
1.0 to 1.5	2.5 to 3	under 25%	35 to 39%
1.5 to 2	3 to 3.5	25 to 29%	40 to 44%
2 to 2.5	3.5 to 4	30 to 34%	45% or more

From Test yourself: how much fat is in your diet? Consumer Reports, p. 393, June 1995.

Assessment 3-3

Name   Section   Date

This is an approximation of the number of Calories your body expands at rest over a 24-hour period. Any activity performed (i.e. walking to class, working out) will require additional energy and also increase total caloric expenditure. How many Calories would you estimate you eat in a given 24-hour period? _____ Calories

Follow the steps below:
1. Go to Figure 3-4. Find your age and then the number of Calories per m^2 per hour. (Fill in 3a below)
2. Go to Figure 3-5. Find your height on Scale I; body mass on Scale II (this is not the middle scale, but on the far right). Lay a ruler or paper on your height at Scale I to your body mass on Scale II; note your "surface area" on the middle Scale III. (Fill in 3b below)
3. To calculate your resting energy expenditure in terms of total Calories, multiply your numbers from 1 and 2 above. Fill in the blanks below.

   a. Number of Calories/m^2 per hour (from Figure 3-4): _____

   b. Surface area (from middle scale in Figure 3-5): _____

   c. (a) _____ × (b) _____ = _____

   d. _____ × 24 hours 5 _____ = Predicted RMR

Example: 55 year old woman. Number of Calories/m^2 per hour = 36; Surface area = 1.4 m^2.

36 Calories × 1.4 m^2 = 50.4 Calories/hour. 50.4 Calories/hour × 24 hours = 1209.6 Calories/24 hours.

4. Your approximate caloric expenditure = _____ Calories (RMR) + 300 Calories

   (daily living) + _____ Calories (workout) = _____ total Calories/day

5. How does this compare to what you think you eat each day? _____

33

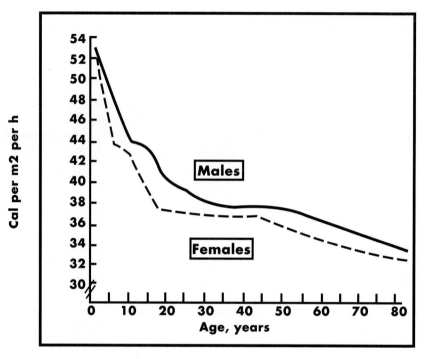

FIGURE 3-4 Basal metabolic rate as a function of age and gender.

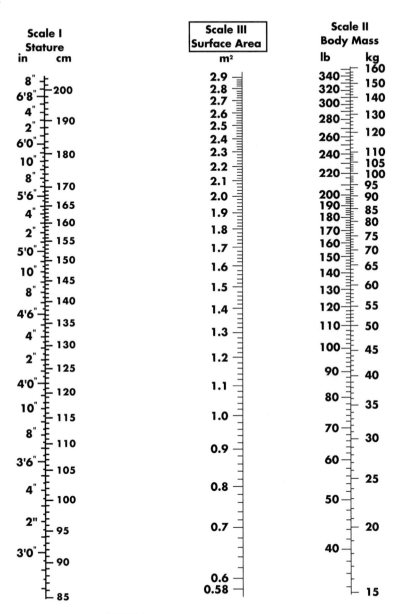

FIGURE 3-5 Basal metabolism nomogram.

Assessment 3-4

Taking the Step Test

Name	Section	Date

To take the step test follow the sequence described below:
1. Use a 12-inch step and a metronome or prerecorded tape set at a cadence of 96 beats per minute.
2. Step up with the right foot, up with the left foot, down with the right foot, then tap the left foot down. The next sequence begins with the left foot: up with the left foot, up with the right, down with the left, then tap down with the right. Continue the up-up-down-down series, alternating the lead leg for 3 minutes at the tempo dictated by the metronome or tape.
3. After 3 minutes of stepping, sit down and find your pulse.
4. Count your recovery heart rate for one full minute and record the number below.
5. Determine your fitness level from the normative values tables below (Table 3-1 and Table 3-2).
6. Retest at the end of the semester, and compare your results. As your fitness level increases, your recovery heart rate should decrease.

Recovery Heart Rate _____

TABLE 3-1
Normative Values for Step Test: Women
Initial Recovery HR:
Fitness Category:

Age (years)	18-25	26-35	36-45	46-55
Excellent	<85	<88	<90	<94
Good	85-98	88-89	90-102	94-104
Above Average	99-108	100-111	103-110	105-115
Average	109-117	112-119	111-118	116-120
Below Average	118-126	120-126	119-128	121-126
Poor	127-140	127-138	129-140	127-135
Very Poor	>140	>138	>140	>135

From Golding LA, Myers CR, and Sinning WE: Y's way to physical fitness, ed. 2, Champaign, Ill, 1989, Human Kinetics Publishers.

TABLE 3-2
Normative Values for Step Test: Men
Initial Recovery HR:
Fitness Category:

Age	18-25	26-35	36-45	46-55
Excellent	<79	<81	<83	<87
Good	79-89	81-89	83-96	87-97
Above average	90-99	90-99	97-103	98-105
Average	100-105	100-107	104-112	106-116
Below Average	106-116	108-117	113-119	117-122
Poor	117-128	118-128	120-130	123-132
Very Poor	>128	>128	>130	>132

From Golding LA, Myers CR, and Sinning WE: Y's way to physical fitness, ed. 2, Champaign, Ill, 1989, Human Kinetics Publishers.

Assessment 3-5

Determining your Body Mass Index

Name   Section   Date

To find your BMI, multiply your weight in pounds by 705, divide that number by your height in inches, and divide that number by your height in inches again.

Example: 140 lb × 705 = 98700 ÷ 64 inches = 1542 ÷ 64 inches = 24.

_____ lb × 705 = _____ ÷ _____ inches = _____ ÷ _____ inches = _____

My BMI is:_____

Note: A BMI of 27.8 or higher for men or 27.3 or higher for women is considered too high and would indicate that you are at risk of health problems related to body weight.

Assessment 3-6

Girth Measurements

Name _____   Section _____   Date _____

Working with a partner, use a measuring tape at the body parts listed in Figure 3-6 below. Record your measurements on the space provided.

Be sure to measure each body part at the largest circumference (widest) or smallest circumference (narrowest) as indicated. Note whether you measure on the right or left side of the body. If possible, measure directly on the skin because clothing will affect your values. Because a change of even ¼ inch is significant, measure as carefully as possible. Try to have the same partner repeat the measurements at the end of the semester.

Body Part	Inches	Right or Left Side
Biceps (widest)		
Chest (widest)		
Waist (narrowest)		
Hips (widest)		
Thigh (widest)		
Calf (widest)		

FIGURE 3-6 Girth Measurement summary log.

Assessment 3-7

Hip Flexibility Test (Flexors and Quadriceps)

Name   Section   Date

This test determines whether there is normal length of the muscles in the front of the hip and thigh. If these muscles are tight, they can cause poor alignment of the lower back and pelvis, causing too much curve in the lower back and too much forward tilt of the pelvis. Too much curve can change the weight distribution in the spine, which can lead to chronic pain and injury. The aim in the test is to keep the back neutral while the thigh rests flat on the table and the knee bends to 90 degrees. Your back is in neutral if the front hip bones and the pubic bone are in the same flat plane.

1. Lie on your back on a table with your knees just past the edge of the table.
2. Lift the left knee until the thigh is slightly past perpendicular to the table, and hold it with your hands. With good flexibility, the right thigh should lie flat on the table with the knee bent and shin vertical (Figure 3-7).
3. If the right thigh is not flat against the table (Figure 3-8), your hip flexors are tight. If the lower leg angles forward, your quadriceps is tight (Figure 3-9).
4. Figures 3-8 and 3-9 show limited hip flexor flexibility. Figure 3-7 shows normal hip flexor flexibility. Compare your position with the figures to assess your flexibility. Circle the appropriate letter (N = normal; L = limited) to record your score below.

Repeat the test with the right knee raised and the left thigh resting against the table.

Left Hip Flexors:	N	L	Right Hip Flexors:	N	L
Left Quadriceps:	N	L	Right Quadriceps	N	L

FIGURE 3-7 Thigh flat on table and shin vertical (normal grade).

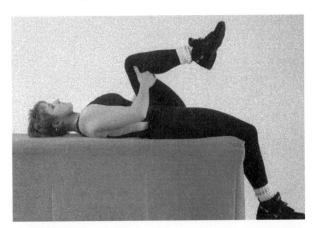

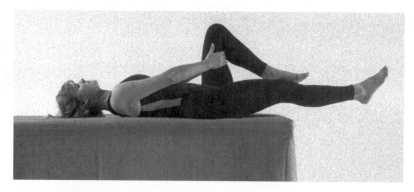

FIGURE 3-8 Limited grade for hip flexor (tight iliopsoas).

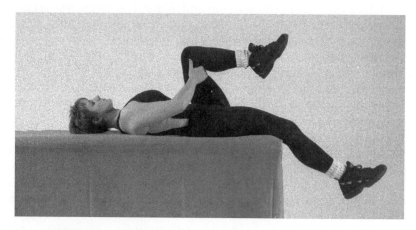

FIGURE 3-9 Limited grade for quadriceps (tight quadriceps).

Assessment 3-8

Knee Flexibility Test (Hamstrings)

Name   Section   Date

Tight hamstrings affect the alignment of your back and pelvis, causing the lower back to be too flat and the pelvis to tilt backward. This can lead to chronic back pain and injury from being out of safe alignment when you are lifting or participating in sports activities.

This test determines whether there is enough flexibility of the hamstring muscles that you can lift your leg with the knee straight, thigh held vertical (perpendicular to the floor). The aim is to be able to keep your hips flat on the floor and one leg straight toward the ceiling.

1. Lie face up on the floor.
2. To assess the right hamstrings, keep the left leg straight against the floor with the hip and knee straight. Do not allow it to bend as you lift the opposite leg. Lift the right leg with the knee straight, as high as possible without allowing the left leg to lift from the floor or table. Keep your hips flat on the floor. For normal range of motion the right (lifted) leg should be perpendicular (85 to 90 degrees) to the floor with the knee straight. The bottom leg must also stay flat against the floor.
3. If you are unable to keep the right knee straight with the leg lifted to 90 degrees, your hamstrings are tight. If the left thigh lifts from the floor, lower the right leg until the left leg is flat and the pelvis is flat (not rolled under).
4. Figure 3-10 shows the various grades of hamstring flexibility. Compare your knee position to the figures. Circle the appropriate letter (N = normal; L = limited; E = excessive) to record your score below.

Repeat the test, raising the left leg.

Left Hamstring: N   L   E
Right Hamstring: N   L   E

Continued

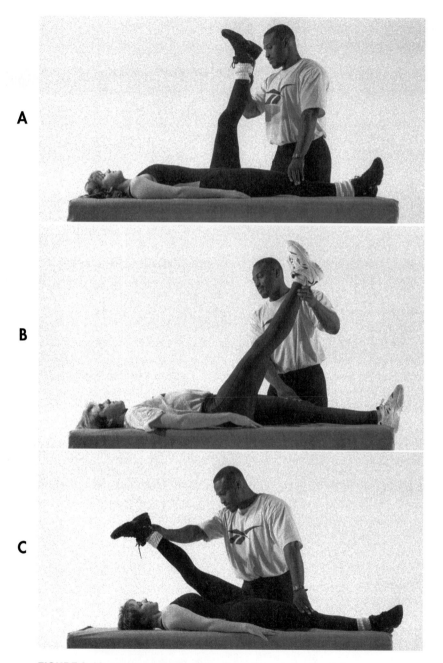

FIGURE 3-10 Grades of hamstring flexibility. A, Normal flexibility (85 to 90 degrees). B, Limited flexibility (less than 85 degrees). C, Excessive flexibility (more than 90 degrees).

Assessment 3-9

Ankle Flexibility Test

Name   Section   Date

Flexibility of the calf muscles is important in body alignment when you are standing. Inflexibility of these muscles or unequal flexibility, right and left, can lead to injury, particularly with impact activities such as running, jogging, aerobic dance, or step aerobics. This test determines the flexibility of the gastrocnemius muscle in your calf. The aim is to be able to pull your forefeet equally away from the board, with the heels touching and the knees straight. Normal range of motion is 20 degrees.

1. Lie face up with your bare feet flat against a wall or a vertical board.
2. Keep your heels in contact with the wall or board. Pull your forefeet away from the wall. Figure 3-11 shows normal ankle flexibility with both sides equal.
3. Check whether your range of motion is equal on both sides. Figure 3-12 shows marked limitation in ankle flexibility. Figure 3-13 shows unequal flexibility. The right side is greater than the left, but both are limited. Have your partner compare your feet with the figures. Circle the appropriate letter (N = normal; L = limited; E = excessive) to record your score below.

Right Calf: N   L   E
Left Calf: N   L   E

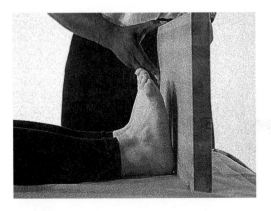

FIGURE 3-11 Normal flexibility of the ankles.

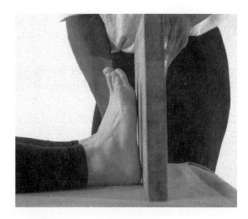

FIGURE 3-12 Limited ankle range of motion.

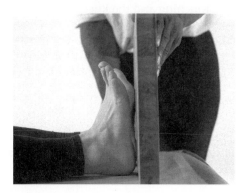

FIGURE 3-13 Limited ankle range of motion, right greater than left.

Assessment 3-10

Shoulder Flexibility Test

Name _____ Section _____ Date _____

Flexibility of the shoulders is important to upper body alignment, especially in overhead activities. If there is limited shoulder range of motion, you may arch the back too much when trying to retrieve something from an overhead position.

This test determines the flexibility of the shoulder and upper body muscles. If tight, these muscles will pull your back and neck out of alignment when you sit or stand and raise your arms overhead. The aim is to keep your back flat on the floor and be able to rest your arms on the floor above your head. If these muscles are tight you need to stretch the chest (pectorals), upper abdominals, and lateral torso (latissimus).

1. Lie face up on the floor with your knees bent and feet flat on the floor. Use your abdominals to keep your back flat on the floor throughout the test. Do not allow your back to arch.

2. With your back flat, lift both arms overhead and place your arms flat on the floor as illustrated in Figure 3-14. Go only as far as you can with your back flat on the floor.

3. Figure 3-15 shows tight shoulders with limited range of motion. Figure 3-16 shows excessive shoulder flexibility. Circle the appropriate letter (N = normal; L = limited; E = excessive) to record your score below.

   Right Shoulder: N   L   E
   Left Shoulder: N   L   E

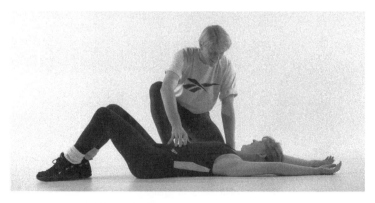

FIGURE 3-14 Shoulder flexibility test.

49

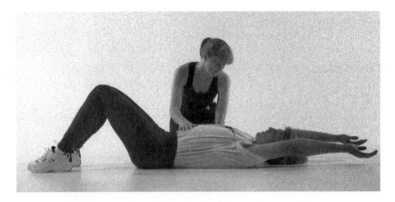

FIGURE 3-15 Limited shoulder range of motion.

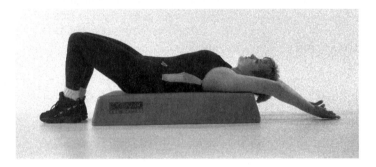

FIGURE 3-16 Excessive shoulder range of motion.

Assessment 3-11

Muscular Strength and Endurance: Push-Up Test

Name   Section   Date

This test requires an ability to stabilize your torso without allowing your head and neck or lower back to sag. It also requires adequate strength in your arms, shoulders, and upper back to lower and lift your own body weight. It is a difficult test. Many people do not have sufficient strength and endurance of their upper body and torso. This test is not graded; the goal is to improve the number of push-ups you can perform over the course of the term.

Figure 3-17 shows excellent push-up form. Many persons have difficulty in performing even one full push-up with perfect form. In that case, modify the movement by performing the bent knee push-up (Figure 3-18). It is essential that you maintain alignment as described and pictured in Figures 3-17 or 3-18. Consistent form now will give you a standard for comparison later; if you try to complete additional push-ups with incorrect form, not only are you increasing your risk of injury, but your future scores will also have less meaning. Note that males have an advantage in this test because more of their mass is concentrated in the upper body and closer to the fulcrum of the movement.

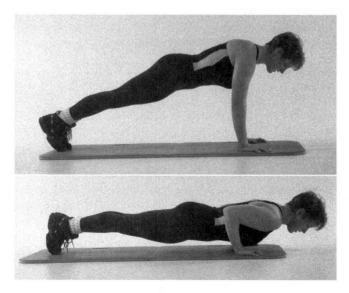

FIGURE 3-17 Excellent form for full push-ups. Maintain this alignment.

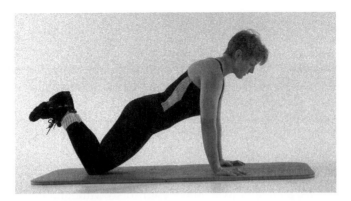

FIGURE 3-18   Bent knee push-up position.

1. Face the floor with your hands under your shoulders and elbows extended. The ankles should be flexed with weight on the balls of the feet (Figure 3-17, A). For the bent-knee version, place the lower body weight just above the knees with the feet lifted (Figure 3-18).
2. Keep your torso and head in a straight line from your heels (or knees) to the base of your skull. Bend the arms and lower the torso until the torso is about 2 inches from the floor, then raise it again by straightening the elbows.
3. Record the number of continuous push-ups (no rests in between) performed with the torso and head perfectly aligned. Do not allow the lower back to sag or lift the buttocks in the air.

Record the number of continuous push-ups (no rests in between) performed with the torso and head perfectly aligned.

Number of push-ups with perfect form _____

Assessment 3-12

Abdominal Stabilization Test (Leg-Lowering Test)

Name   Section   Date

There are two types of abdominal tests: the regular sit-up test, which looks at your ability to flex the torso as many times as possible in a minute, and the leg-lowering test, which looks at your ability to stabilize the torso (hold it still against the floor), resisting the action of the legs (weight and the contraction of the hip muscles), which tends to lift the back from the floor.

In the leg lowering test, the abdominals must be strong enough to maintain control of the pelvis and keep the back down. It is a difficult test, but an important one in assessing your ability to stabilize your back during activities such as lifting heavy objects. The aim is to hold the lower back flat on the table or floor while slowly lowering both legs from the vertical.

1. Lie face up on the floor with your arms crossed on your chest or behind your head. Lift your legs one at a time to a vertical position. Your partner places one hand at the edge of your lower back with the fingers at the edge of the sacrum, and the other hand beneath (but not holding) your legs (Figure 3-19).

2. Contract your abdominal muscles to press your back flat on the floor and put pressure on the partner's fingers under the back. Slowly lower both legs to the floor with the knees straight, focusing on maintaining a strong abdominal contraction to keep the back flat and pressure on the partner's fingers. Do not raise the head or shoulders during the test.

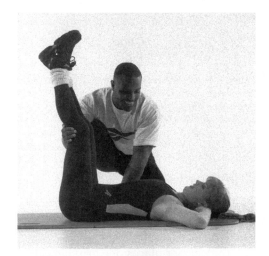

FIGURE 3-19 Abdominal stabilization test. Partner places one hand at the edge of your lower back with fingers at the edge of the sacrum, the other hand beneath (but not holding) your legs.

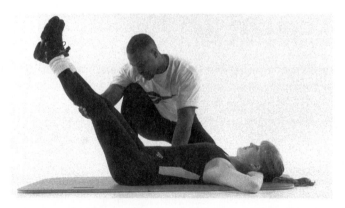

FIGURE 3-20 Abdominal stabilization test. Partner places one arm beneath your legs as they lower to the floor. Check angle of legs with the floor when the back begins to lift from the floor.

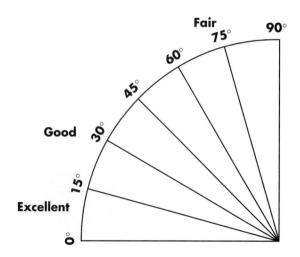

FIGURE 3-21 Abdominal stabilization test. Partner should compare your leg positions with the angle in the diagram to grade the strength of your torso stabilizers.

The partner places one arm beneath your legs as they lower toward the floor (Figure 3-20).

3. When your back begins to lift from the floor (releasing pressure from the partner's fingers), your partner should support your legs. Your partner then compares your leg position with Figure 3-21 to grade the strength of the torso stabilizers. Figure 3-22 shows excellent abdominal stabilizing strength, with the back held flat as the legs lower to about 15 degrees.

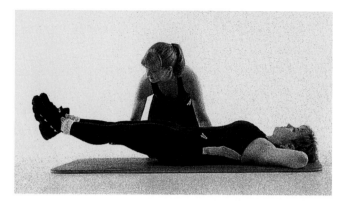

FIGURE 3-22   Excellent abdominal stabilization strength.

The need for stabilizing your torso in neutral is particularly important when you sit much of the day: in class, driving, working at a desk. In the sitting position, the ligaments of your hips and pelvis cannot help with the support because the hips are flexed. In standing, with the hips straight, you can "lean" on the ligaments to stay upright. In sitting these ligaments are "slack" so you must rely on muscular endurance to maintain that support. Males should grade excellent; females should grade good. Males have an slight advantage in this test, because less of their mass is in their legs.

If you grade only fair in this test, work on stabilization exercises for the abdominal muscles (see Chapter 12).

Abdominal stabilization strength: Fair _____ Good _____ Excellent _____

Assessment 3-13

Postural Assessment

Name   Section   Date

Neutral alignment of your back and joints not only looks better but also prevents many of the chronic aches and pains that people experience every day. The ability to hold your body securely in safe alignment may prevent many of the injuries that occur in sports and everyday tasks such as lifting and moving heavy loads.

Functional alignment of the body is difficult when muscles are out of balance, with some muscles too tight and some muscles too weak. If your scores on the muscular strength and endurance tests are less than ideal, you can expect that your alignment will be less than ideal. Even if you can achieve good alignment during the assessment, the crucial question is whether you have the strength, endurance and flexibility to *maintain* that alignment throughout the day during your daily activities.

Check your partner's alignment from the front, side, and back to get a complete picture. Compare the specific landmarks of the body to a plumb line to understand what you are seeing. The plumb line in Figure 3-23 is a piece of string with a small weight at the end, attached to the ceiling or the top of a door frame. It makes a perfectly straight vertical line that serves as a basis of comparison.

Continued on p. 58.

FRONT VIEW

To check the front view, position your partner's body so that the base of the plumb line falls halfway between the feet. Check for straight ankles, kneecaps facing forward at the same level, even hip bones, even shoulders, and straight (not tilted) head (Figure 3-23).

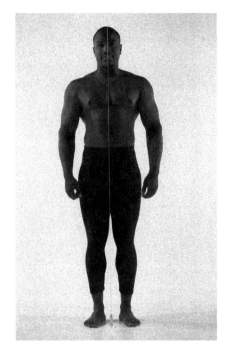

FIGURE 3-23 Postural assessment, front view.

Circle those items that apply:

	Poorly Aligned	**Centered**	**Poorly Aligned**
Plumb Line Falls			
Ankles	Tilted in	Even	Tilted out
Knee Caps	Left higher	Even	Right higher
	Face in	Face forward	Face outward
Knees	Bow in	Parallel	Bow out
Hips	Left higher	Even	Right higher
Shoulders	Left higher	Even	Right high
Head	Tilted left	Straight	Tilted right

SIDE VIEW

To check the side, the base of the plumb line should fall just in front of the ankle bone. Check for a slight inward curve of the lower back, flat abdomen, lifted chest, and that the back of the hand faces the side. The plumb line should pass just behind the kneecap and through the middle of the hip joint, shoulder, and ear canal (Figure 3-24).

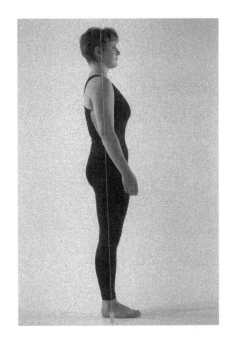

FIGURE 3-24 Postural assessment, side view.

Circle those items that apply:

	Poorly Aligned	**Centered**	**Poorly Aligned**
Plumb Line Falls	Far behind kneecap	Just behind kneecap	Through kneecap
Plumb Line Falls	Behind hip	Through center of hip	In front of hip
Plumb Line Falls	Behind shoulder	Through center of shoulder	In front of shoulder
Plumb Line Falls	Behind ear	Through center of ear	In front of ear
Back of Hand	Faces forward	Faces side	
Lower Back	Flat	Slight inward curve	Large inward curve
Abdomen		Flat	Protruding
Chest	Collapsed	Lifted over instep	

BACK VIEW

Position your partner so that the bottom of the plumb line falls midway between the heels. The plumb line should fall so that the body is split into equal halves, right and left, through the center of the buttocks, center of the spine and the center of the head. The Achilles tendons should be vertical (not bowed in or out). The folds behind the knee should be at the same level on both sides. The hips and shoulders should be level. The head should be straight, not tilted. The shoulder blades should be level and flat on the back, about 2 inches on either side of the spine (Figure 3-25).

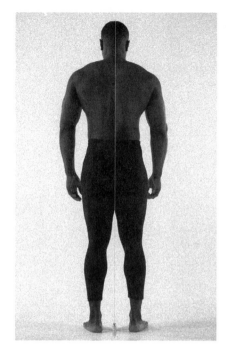

FIGURE 3-25 Postural assessment, back view.

Circle those items that apply:

	Poorly Aligned	**Centered**	**Poorly Aligned**
Plumb Line Falls	To the left	Through the center of the buttock	To the right
Plumb Line Falls	To the left	Through the center of the spine	To the right
Plumb Line Falls	To the left	Through the center of the head	To the right
Achilles Tendons	Bow inward	Are vertical	Bow outward
Knee folds	Left are higher	Even	Right are higher
Hips	Left is higher	Even	Right is higher
Shoulders	Left is higher	Even	Right is higher

Continued

	Poorly Aligned	Centered	Poorly Aligned
Shoulder Blades	Left is more than 2 inches from the spine	Both about 2 inches from the spine	Right is more than 2 inches from the spine
Shoulder Blades	Left is higher	Even	Right is higher
Head	Tilted left	Straight	Tilted right

The postural assessment has no score, but it would be helpful to reassess your posture at mid-term and final to note any improvements in your overall alignment.

A balanced exercise program of strength, endurance, and flexibility will help you balance your body and bring it into a functional, neutral alignment. However, endurance in neutral alignment can be developed only by consciously realigning yourself whenever you notice yourself sitting or standing incorrectly. That is up to you throughout the day.

FITNESS ASSESSMENT SUMMARY

Record your scores from each of the previous tests on this form.

	BASELINE	MID-TERM	FINAL

Aerobic Fitness
  Recovery HR
  (Assessment 3-4)			

BMI (Assessment 3-5)			
Girth Measurements			
Biceps			
Chest			
Waist			
Thigh			
Calf (Assessment 3-6)			
Flexibility			
Hip Flexors R/L (Assessment 3-7)			
Hamstrings R/L (Assessment 3-8)			
Ankles/Calf muscles R/L (Assessment 3-9)			
Shoulders R/L (Assessment 3-10)			
Strength/Endurance			

No. of push ups
  (note full or bent knee)
  (Assessment 3-11)			

Abdominals/leg lowering (Assessment 3-12)			

Summary Worksheet for Self-Assessment

Assessment	Measurement	Baseline	Mid-term	Final
3-1 PAR-Q & You	Physical readiness for activity without a doctor's consent:			
Health risk appraisal	Range of physical activity participation (none; light to moderate; vigorous; resistance training):			
	Working for positive active life style changes:			
	Consume a healthy diet:			
3-2 Test yourself: how much fat is in your diet?	Percent of Calories from fat:			
3-3 Estimating your basal metabolic rate	Caloric intake:			
	Caloric expenditure:			
3-4 Taking the step test	Recovery heart rate:			
3-5 Determining your body mass index	BMI:			

Summary Worksheet for Self-Assessment—cont'd

Assessment	Measurement	Baseline	Mid-term	Final
3-6 Girth Measurements	Biceps:			
	Chest:			
	Waist:			
	Thigh:			
	Calf:			
3-7 Hip Flexibility Test	Hip flexors R/L:			
3-8 Knee Flexibility Test	Hamstrings:			
3-9 Ankle Flexibility Test	Ankles/Calf muscles R/L:			
3-10 Shoulder Flexibility Test	Shoulders R/L			
3-11 Push-up Test	Number of push-ups (note full or bent knee):			
3-12 Abdominal Stabilization Test	Abdominals/leg lowering (F, G, E):			
3-13 Postural Assessment	Notes on overall alignment:			

CHAPTER 4

DEVELOPING THE **BIG PICTURE:** THE ACTION PLAN

OBJECTIVES

After reading this chapter, you should be able to do the following:

- Set realistic goals toward improving your level of fitness and determine a plan of action that is right for you.
- List the components of a complete fitness program and explain their importance.

KEY TERMS

While reading this chapter, you will become familiar with the following terms:

▶ Action Plan
▶ Maintenance

▶ Personal Goals

PUTTING IT ALL TOGETHER

Now that you have gotten an initial picture of your current overall fitness level with the screening assessment tools provided in Chapter 3, it is time to determine whether you want to make some changes in how the picture is shaping up. Setting **personal goals** with an **action plan** to help you achieve those goals will help you maximize your time and effort. In the same way that a box cover serves as a guide to putting together a puzzle, your personal goals can identify your overall purpose (the big picture), and the action plan can help you put the individual pieces together. In addition, by looking at each of the pieces of the puzzle separately, you can begin to see where they fit together and how they differ, to ensure that you are developing a complete program. You will first set goals and an accompanying action plan. Then you will follow through on the steps you have identified as necessary to accomplish your goals.

GOAL SETTING

Goals should be specific and measurable, according to a plan of action with a predetermined deadline. A specific goal is focused. You should identify the target, and your action plan should reflect your desire to hit the bull's-eye. By linking a plan of action (e.g., "I will work out four times a week for 12 weeks and then maintain with three workouts a week") with your goals (reduce recovery heart rate after the step test by 10 beats per minute) you can more easily measure progress. Nebulous, intangible goals (e.g., "I want to feel better") are difficult to quantify, yielding little satisfaction because it is difficult to determine what you have accomplished. Setting both short- and long-term goals with deadlines to evaluate your progress can create a sense of ownership and personal investment that will help you stick with your program. You may want to partner with someone for encouragement and accountability. Sharing your goals with someone may give you both added incentive to achieve them.

▶ Keep Them Within Reach

Most importantly, your goals should be realistic. You should honestly consider whether it is possible to achieve a particular goal over the allotted time period. Individual goals should be just that: realistic for you, not for a large group or several friends. If you are just beginning to exercise, for instance, it is unlikely that you would reach a goal of qualifying for the Boston Marathon by the end of 4 months, although you might complete a 5K or 10K walk or run. In addition, realistic goal setting requires that you have the ability to bring about the desired change. Many persons begin an exercise program with unrealistic expectations and unachievable goals because they have been affected by societal norms that deem one "look" to be better or more acceptable than another. An unreachable goal

Goal Setting Worksheet

Name _____   Section _____   Date _____

	Mid-term Date_____	Final Date_____
HRA: Physical Activity		
Goal		
Benefits		
Actions		
Key Resources		
Measurements		

▶ Physical Activity Goals

Because you are involved in aerobic dance exercise on a regular basis, you might look at ways to become more active throughout the day (e.g., take the stairs rather than the elevator at least once a day). Consider adding some form of resistance training twice a week and possibly trying a new or different activity, such as yoga.

Goal Setting Worksheet

Name   Section   Date

	Mid-term Date_____	Final Date_____
HRA: Lifestyle		
Goal		
Benefits		
Actions		
Key Resources		
Measurements		

▶ Lifestyle Goals

If you answered "yes" to any of the questions in the lifestyle section of the HRA, determine if this behavior creates personal problems or difficulties in your relationships with others. If so, you might want to begin to alter your behavior, but you should recognize that some habits are easier to change than others. Although it might be relatively easy to decide to start wearing sunscreen, stopping smoking could be much more difficult. The first step is to identify an area in which you would like to see change, then determine if you can make the change yourself or if you might need some professional assistance.

Goal Setting Worksheet

Name   Section   Date

	Mid-term Date_____	**Final** Date_____
HRA: Dietary and Fat Intake		
Goal		
Benefits		
Actions		
Key Resources		
Measurement		

▶ Dietary and Fat Intake Goals

Ideally your diet should be high in complex carbohydrates (58% or more), with only about 25% to 30% of your calories coming from fat and about 12% from protein. Often fat is hidden in processed or prepared foods, and it can be difficult to be certain how much fat you are consuming. If your dietary fat intake is high, try to reduce that percentage by at least one category by the end of the semester (about a 5% reduction). Although there are many ways to accomplish this, one way would be to limit your consumption of red meat or high- fat cuts of meat. You could also reduce your intake of full-fat dairy products, substituting low-fat or skim products whenever possible.

Exercise is most effective when it is combined with a balanced, nutrient-dense diet that is adequate in calories and low in fat and simple sugars. Increasing your intake of fruits, grains, and vegetables can affect your overall health by providing more energy and even reducing your risk of developing certain cancers. Adequate levels of dietary calcium are of particular importance for women, who are at greater risk of developing osteoporosis, or bone loss. Additional information on diet and exercise is available in Chapters 6 and 7.

Goal Setting Worksheet

Name _____ Section _____ Date _____

	Mid-term Date_____	Final Date_____
Aerobic Fitness		
Goal		
Benefits		
Actions		
Key Resources		
Measurements		

▶ AEROBIC FITNESS GOALS

Your initial fitness level at the time you start with this class will be directly linked with how much you can expect to improve. If you begin in the *good* category of Table 3-1 or 3-2, it may take the entire semester or even longer to move into the *excellent* category. If you start out the semester at a low level of fitness, though, you can expect to improve by at least one category by the mid-term and potentially another or even more by the final assessment.

Example: You might start with a recovery heart rate of 137, which is at the low end of the *poor* category. A reasonable mid-term goal would be a recovery heart rate of 118 (at the top of the *average* category) with a final goal of 106, which moves you into the *above average* category.

Goal Setting Worksheet

Name   Section   Date

	Mid-term Date_____	**Final** Date_____
Body Composition and Girth Measurements		
Goal		
Benefits		
Actions		
Key Resources		
Measurements		

▶ GIRTH MEASUREMENT GOALS

Even small changes in body size can be significant. If you decrease a girth measurement by ¼ to ½ inch, that is tremendous progress! If you increase a measurement by ¼ to ½ inch, you have potentially gained some muscle mass. Because of the sensitivity of these measurements, be sure you work carefully and try to have the same partner working with you during each assessment.

Goal Setting Worksheet

Name   Section   Date

	Mid-term Date_____	**Final Date_____**
Flexibility		
Goal		
Benefits		
Actions		
Key Resources		
Measurements		

▶ FLEXIBILITY GOALS

Because your flexibility may vary from joint to joint, you may want to set more than one flexibility goal, each joint-specific. If you found limitations (*L* grade on the assessments), focus on those specific areas in your flexibility training plan. If you found that your range of motion is excessive (*E* on assessment) in some areas, concentrate on building strength in those muscle groups. This is particularly true if you have a problem with hyperextension of the knees or elbows.

A reasonable goal would be to move from limited to normal range of motion over the course of the term. Again, be specific in goal-setting and time spent stretching: for example, you may need to concentrate on the right shoulder or the left hamstring, not just general, overall stretching. Remember that stretching must be performed *daily* for noticeable progress to occur.

Goal Setting Worksheet

Name   Section   Date

	Mid-term Date_____	**Final** Date_____
Muscular Strength and Endurance		
Goal		
Benefits		
Actions		
Key Resources		
Measurements		

MUSCULAR STRENGTH AND ENDURANCE GOALS

▶ Push-ups

Many people are initially unable to complete even one push-up with correct form. As we stated previously, a perfectly executed push-up requires significant upper body strength as well as muscular strength to stabilize the torso. If you performed the test with bent knees but completed less than 10 repetitions, a reasonable goal would be to perform 20 to 30 bent-knee push-ups by mid-term and perhaps 5 to 10 full push-ups by the end of the term.

▶ Abdominals

The possible grades on the abdominal stabilization tests were *fair* (F), *good* (G), and *excellent* (E). For a healthy back and abdominal strength, men should grade *excellent*. Women should be able to achieve at least a grade of *good* by the end of the term. If your score was *fair*, it would be reasonable to increase by one category by mid-term and another grade by the end of the term.

Men have a slight advantage in this test because more of their mass is concentrated in the upper body, while women have more mass in the lower body. The test uses the weight of the lower body as resistance, so that women are potentially working against a proportionally greater resistance.

Goal Setting Worksheet

Name   Section   Date

	Mid-term Date_____	Final Date_____
Posture		
Goal		
Benefits		
Actions		
Key Resources		
Measurements		

▶ POSTURAL GOALS

The goals in this area may be as simple as being centered in 80% of the areas examined from the side, front, or back in the next assessment at mid-term or final. If you have a specific problem area that one of the tests identifies, you might set a goal to ask your instructor or trainer for specific advice or training tips to improve that area.

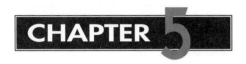

CHAPTER 5

YOUR ACTION PLAN: A POSITIVE START

OBJECTIVES

After reading this chapter, you should be able to do the following:

- Understand the importance of proper apparel, hydration, working out at the proper intensity, rest and recovery, and the possible warning signs of injury.
- Be aware of exercises with a risk of injury and modify those so that you can safely participate in classes that contain exercises with a known high risk of injury.

KEY TERMS

While reading this chapter, you will become familiar with the following terms:

▶ Overuse Injuries   ▶ RICE

UNDERSTANDING IMPACT AND AVOIDING OVERUSE INJURIES

Most injuries sustained in dance-exercise classes are classified as **overuse injuries**. Overuse injuries result from repeated stresses to a particular body part that is not prepared—because of inadequate strength, endurance, or flexibility or inadequate rest or recovery time—to handle the stress. Such injuries can be avoided with certain precautions that allow the muscles, tendons, ligaments, and bones to adapt gradually to the increased mechanical stresses.

The following are guidelines for reducing the risk of overuse injuries. Keep them in mind as you begin your exercise program. Do not rush the process of getting in shape; your body must have the time necessary to get stronger and adapt to the increased demands of vigorous activity. Staying injury free is an important part of enjoying your fitness program and staying motivated to continue it.

SHOES AND APPAREL

Choose shoes with adequate stability and cushioning for shock absorption, traction, and support for the up-and-down and side-to-side movements of a dance-exercise class. The forefoot should have more cushioning for dance exercise because you land on the ball of the foot in these movements. The heel should have more cushioning for an activity such as jogging, because the impact is at the heel. Therefore, running shoes are not ideally suited for dance exercise, and shoes designed for dance exercise are not the best choice for jogging.

Choose apparel appropriate for the environmental conditions. Wear clothing that allows unrestricted blood flow to all body parts and evaporation of perspiration for proper regulation of body temperature. Light-weight, cotton fabrics are cooler than synthetic fabrics, which tend to retain heat.

Never wear plastic or nonbreathable clothing while exercising. The idea that increased sweating will increase fat loss is a dangerous myth. The evaporation of sweat is an important mechanism to keep your body from overheating.

It is also helpful to plan ahead with a specific bag or locker to keep necessary equipment, shoes, and apparel at hand. Otherwise, it is easy to forget something and use that as an excuse for not working out or not being able to work out because you forgot your shoes.

PROPER HYDRATION

Normally people rely on the sensation of thirst as a cue to drink water and how much to drink. However, during exercise thirst may not be an accurate indication of the body's need for water. Internal fluid levels are particularly important during exercise, because fluid in blood and tissues transports nutrients and waste-products to and away from muscles. In addition, fluid in sweat helps to regulate body temperature.

Drinking from 4 to 8 ounces of water every 10 to 20 minutes during vigorous exercise is recommended to replace fluid losses. In hot, humid weather the losses can be even greater and additional hydration before exercise (hyperhydration) may help prepare for the added heat stress. If you wish to hyperhydrate in hot, humid weather, the recommendation is to drink 2 to 3 cups of water 2 to 3 hours before exercise and then 1 to 2 cups about 1½ hours before.

Cool water is the drink for exercisers. It empties from the stomach rapidly and is quickly absorbed by the body. Drinks containing sugar, such as soft drinks and some sport drinks, take longer to be absorbed.

PROPER PROGRESSION AND INTENSITY

Come to class on time, so that you use the warm-up period to prepare your body for the more vigorous activity levels of the training session. Sufficient warm-up enhances the metabolic processes and prevents injury.

Begin exercising at an intensity appropriate for your present level of fitness. Your instructor should present movement choices of various intensities; choose a lower or moderate intensity initially if you are just beginning an exercise program. Injuries can occur if you attempt to workout at too high a level too quickly.

Progress slowly and make only one change at a time. Do not increase the frequency, intensity, and duration of exercise all at the same time. Give your body time to adapt to the new stresses on the heart, lungs, muscles, connective tissue, and bones. If you progress too fast and train more frequently than your body can recover, you may sustain an overuse injury (many of which are described later in Table 5-1).

Your body's ability to participate safely in vigorous activity may vary slightly from time to time. It is possible to exercise too hard during a session. If during exercise you experience dizziness, nausea, shortness of breath, high heart rate, extreme fatigue, or tightness in your chest, you are exercising too hard. Stop immediately and consult your instructor.

SUFFICIENT REST AND RECOVERY

Get adequate rest between classes. Your body needs sufficient time to recover between exercise sessions. Overtraining can be as harmful to your health as not training. Some signals of overtraining include inability to sleep, fatigue, and a resting heart rate that is higher than normal.

STOP AND PAY ATTENTION TO PAIN

Pay attention to your body and any signs of pain or ongoing discomfort. Mild muscle soreness can be expected initially with vigorous exercise. However joint, bone, or severe muscle pain is not to be expected; if it occurs, it is your body's signal

▶ **Overuse Injuries**
Avoidable injuries caused by repeated stress to a particular body part with inadequate rest and recovery.

to you that something is wrong. Discontinue exercises that cause undue discomfort. Do not try to "work through" an injury. Stop the activity, and consult a physician if necessary. If swelling or discomfort persists past 48 hours, seek medical attention.

MODIFY HIGHER-RISK EXERCISES FOR SAFETY

Be aware of the potential risks of certain exercises, and adapt movements to avoid possible injury. Several common exercises that are possible safety risks are pictured in this section along with modifications for improved safety technique.

These higher-risk exercises are presented so that you are aware of why they are not being used in this class. Modifications are suggested so that if you encounter them in another class or at your health club, you will know safe alternatives.

WINDMILL OR BOUNCING WITH THE BACK FLEXED FORWARD

Fast, bouncing, or many repeated forward bends of the lower back can place the ligaments and discs of the spine at risk. Opposite toe-touches and bouncing while bending forward at the waist can place undesirable stress on the lower back, especially if one has been sitting all day with the back rounded forward. If an exercise calls for a forward bend, bend from the hips instead of the lower back. When you bend from the hips, your back should retain its normal inward curve (the back muscles are contracting, not relaxed).

Unsupported flexion of the back is particularly a problem if bouncing, fast, or repeated movements are done in this position (Figure 5-1). Opposite toe-touches (Figure 5-2) are also not recommended. Figure 5-3 illustrates a recommended modification for safe hamstring stretch with hip joints flexing forward and lower back in neutral (neutral is in the middle, neither flexed nor hyperextended).

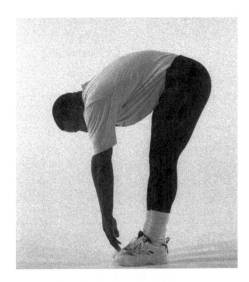

FIGURE 5-1 Unsupported flexion of the back is a problem if bouncing or repeated movements are done in this position.

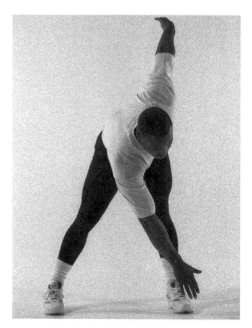

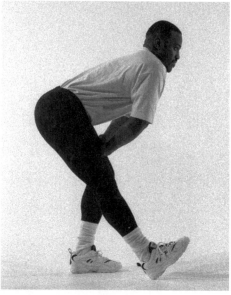

FIGURE 5-2 Opposite toe-touches (windmill) are not recommended.

FIGURE 5-3 Recommended modification for safe hamstring stretch with back in neutral position.

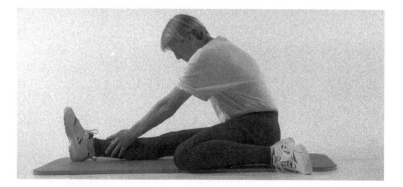

FIGURE 5-4 The traditional hamstring hurdler's stretch is not recommended.

HURDLER STRETCHES

Hurdler stretches have been used traditionally to stretch the hamstrings (Figure 5-4) and quadriceps (Figure 5-5). If performed improperly they may overstretch the ligament along the inside of the knee joint. This ligament is important for knee support and, once overstretched, will not provide the necessary support.

Figure 5-6 shows an alternate hamstring stretch. Figure 5-7 shows an alternate stretch for the quadriceps.

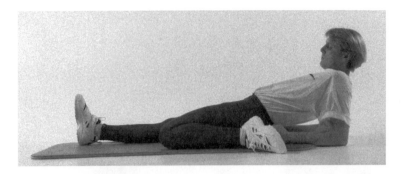

FIGURE 5-5 The traditional quadriceps hurdler's stretch is not recommended.

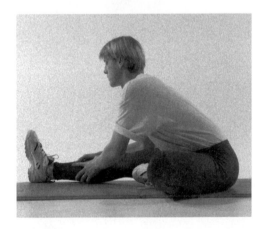

FIGURE 5-6 Recommended modification for safe hamstring stretch.

FIGURE 5-7 Recommended modification for safe quadriceps stretch.

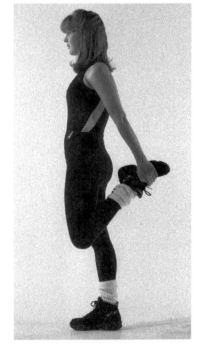

PLOUGH

The plough (Figure 5-8) is sometimes used to stretch the back. Although this exercise can be performed safely, it requires considerable flexibility of the legs and spine as well as excellent motor control. Improper technique can place excessive stress on the spine of the upper back and neck, especially if you are not flexible and if your neck muscles are not strong.

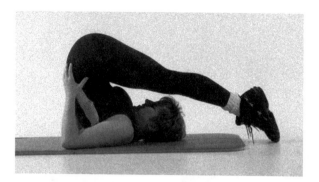

FIGURE 5-8 Plough may put neck at risk.

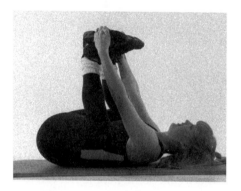

FIGURE 5-9 Alternative lower back stretch.

Figure 5-9 shows a safe stretch for the lower back. Hold the feet and press the knees straight toward the floor. The flexing of the hips will provide a stretch to the deep lower back muscles. Lift your head to increase the stretch along all the muscles along the spine.

FAST CIRCLING

Fast circling of any joint, but particularly the neck or spine, could result in a serious injury. With high-speed movements, the forces involved with the momentum must be absorbed by the ligaments. The ligaments as well as the internal structures of the joints can be damaged when movement is not under muscular control. Therefore head rolls or neck rolls are less risky if performed in 4 segments: flex to the right shoulder, then return to the center, look up toward the ceiling then back to the center, flex toward the left shoulder, then back to the center, chin to the chest, then back to the center.

JOINT HYPEREXTENSION WITH RESISTANCE

Ligaments, which connect bone to bone, are important in stabilizing the joints and in preventing undesirable motion. For example, you do not want your knees to bend from side to side, so there are strong ligaments on the inside and outside of the knee to prevent those motions. Some people seem to have loose ligaments behind their knees or in front of their elbows that allow those joints to extend too

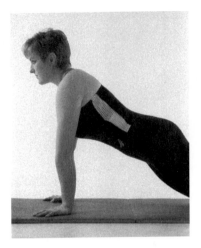

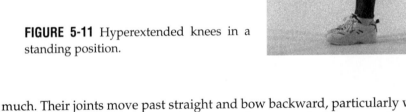

FIGURE 5-10 Hyperextended elbows in a push-up position.

FIGURE 5-11 Hyperextended knees in a standing position.

much. Their joints move past straight and bow backward, particularly when bearing weight and when the supporting muscles are weak. Some people refer to this condition as "locking out" the joints.

Figure 5-10 shows hyperextended elbows in a push-up position. Figure 5-11 shows slightly hyperextended knees in the standing position. Repeated hyperextension can cause continued stretching of the ligaments and undesirable stress on the surfaces of the joints.

People who tend to hyperextend should work to develop increased muscular strength around those joints to provide stabilization of the involved joints by the muscles. They should also continuously check their joint position in a mirror, instead of going by how their body feels. If they hyperextend normally, the hyperextended position will feel "right." The correct neutral joint position will *feel* slightly flexed to the hyperextended person, even though it is not.

The joints that seem more vulnerable to hyperextended positions are the wrists, elbows, and knees. Past the neutral position (neutral is in the middle, neither flexed nor hyperextended), the ligaments may overstretch, particularly if the movement is performed repeatedly or with resistance such as weights or elastic. Overstretched ligaments can make the joint less stable. Figures 5-12 and 5-13 are two additional examples of joint hyperextension that can make you more prone to injury.

Another time that hyperextension may be a problem is when elastic resistance (bands or tubing) is held in the hands (Figures 5-14 and 5-15). Take care to monitor the position of the wrists when using elastic. Make sure the wrists are straight, not cocked backward.

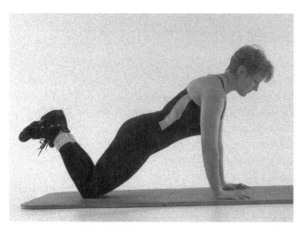

FIGURE 5-12 "Soft" elbows in the up-phase of the push-up.

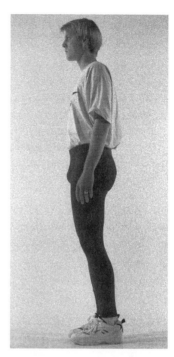

FIGURE 5-13 "Soft" extension of knees.

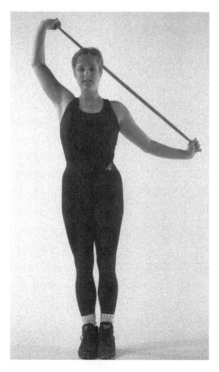

FIGURE 5-14 Hyperextended wrists with elastic band.

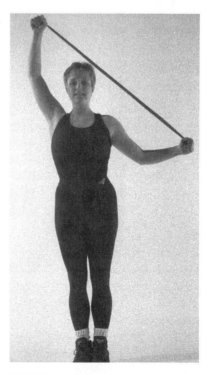

FIGURE 5-15 Neutral wrists with elastic band.

DOUBLE LEG LOWERING

Holding the back stable while lowering both extended legs is a very difficult exercise, requiring excellent strength of the abdominal muscles. It is a test position (see Chapter 3) but is not advisable as an initial training technique. Often the muscles of the hips and pelvis are unbalanced. When weakness and imbalance are present, repeating this movement as an exercise can cause a strain to the lower back.

Your abdominal work should progress very carefully. Begin stabilization training with the knees bent and alternate lowering the right leg, then the left. The next step might be to lower both legs with the knees bent. Master stabilization with lower resistance (knees bent) before attempting it with higher levels of resistance. Figure 5-16 shows a stabilization exercise with moderate resistance, and Figure 5-17 illustrates an action that is not recommended if you have inadequate abdominal strength.

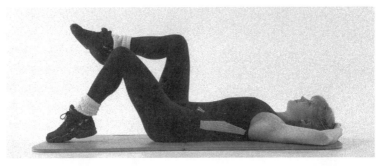

FIGURE 5-16 Stabilization with moderate resistance (alternate toe tap). Use abdominals to keep back on the floor.

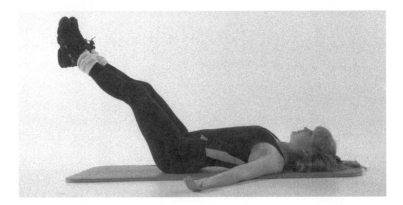

FIGURE 5-17 Lowering straight legs with inadequate abdominal strength may cause lower back strain. Notice that lower back lifts off the floor showing poor abdominal control. This is not recommended as an exercise for beginners.

STRAIGHT LEG FULL SIT-UPS

In performing straight leg sit-ups (Figure 5-18), many people use momentum and the strength of the hip flexors to pop their torso to the upright position. Repeated use of this technique may make an existing muscle imbalance even worse, because it strengthens the hip flexors, while the abdominals remain weaker. The need is to strengthen the abdominals to make them more equal with the hip flexors. The modification (Figure 5-19) causes you to use the lower abdominals to press the back down and the upper abdominals to lift the shoulders. The hip flexors are not as active in the modified position, so muscular balance can be achieved. Try and keep the gluteals relaxed during this activity.

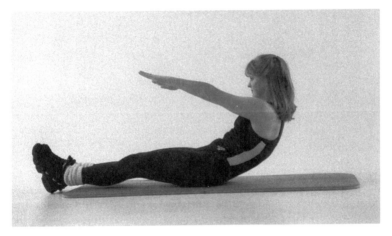

FIGURE 5-18 Straight leg sit-ups are not recommended.

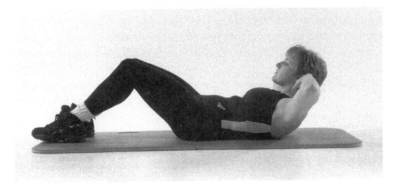

FIGURE 5-19 Tilt and curls: flatten the back using the abdominals, then lift the upper torso.

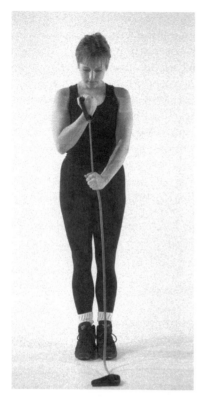

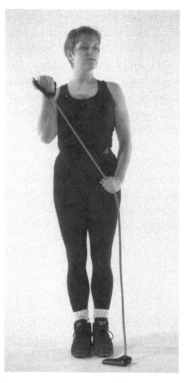

FIGURE 5-20 A line of pull near the eyes (elastic line pull) is not recommended.

FIGURE 5-21 Safe alternative: same exercise as in Figure 5-20, but with a diagonal anchor point and the participant looking in another direction.

ELASTIC LINE OF PULL NEAR FACE

Always check elastic resistance bands before each use for signs of wear or fraying. Never use worn or defective products, because the elastic could tear and hit you or another person nearby in the face or eyes. Make sure the line of pull does not go near your eyes. Modify the anchor point and your gaze to protect your eyes.

Figure 5-20 shows a line of pull near the eyes and the participant looking toward the elastic. Figure 5-21 shows the same exercise with a diagonal anchor point and the participant looking in another direction.

COMMON OVERUSE INJURIES IN DANCE EXERCISE

Most injuries in dance exercise occur to the lower part of the body or to the shoulder joint. Table 5-1 summarizes, in alphabetical order, the most common conditions, symptoms, possible causes, and guidelines for prevention and treatment. If you are injured, stop the activity and let your instructor know immediately.

RICE is the usually recommended treatment for a minor injury. It is an acronym that stands for *rest, ice,* compression (wrapping), and *elevation.*

▶ **RICE**
Initial first-aid technique for treating injuries; includes *rest, ice,* compression, and *elevation.*

SUMMARY

- Staying injury free is an important part of enjoying and staying motivated to continue your fitness program.
- Proper apparel, hydration, progression, and intensity, sufficient rest and recovery, and paying attention to pain are essential for maximizing the long-term results of your fitness program.
- You should modify high-risk activities to decease your chances of injury. Pay attention to your body and stop if you experience pain or discomfort while performing an exercise.
- If you become injured while exercising, stop the activity and let your instructor know immediately. RICE is usually the recommended treatment for a minor injury.
- Proper initial care of an injury will decrease your pain, discomfort, and recovery time.

TABLE 5-1
Overuse Injuries, Conditions, Symptoms, Causes, Prevention and Treatment

Injury	Symptoms	Possible cause	Prevention/Medical treatment (℞)
Achilles tendinitis— Inflammation of the tendon attaching the calf muscles to the heel	Tenderness to touch over the Achilles tendon; pain when the ankle is flexed	Inadequate warm-up before impact activity; inadequate calf flexibility	Adequate warm-up; regular calf stretching ℞: Rest, ice affected area, mild stretching; limit activity if symptoms worsen
Ankle sprain— Overstretching or tearing ankle ligaments, usually on the outside of the joint	Pain, swelling, discoloration over the affected ligament; limited range of motion of the ankle	Extreme inward movement of the ankle beyond the normal range of motion; traction between shoes and carpeted surface	Match shoes to floor surface ℞: Limit weight-bearing uneven floor surface; too much activity; RICE immediately and for 48-72 hours; consult a physician to rule out fracture
Biceps tendinitis— Inflammation of the tendon of the biceps as it crosses the shoulder	Pain and tenderness to touch in front of the shoulder joint; pain may increase with resisted contraction of the biceps	Fast pumping movements of the arms, particularly with the elbows extended	Decrease tempo of arm movements; perform them half-time or with elbows bent ℞: Rest; ice affected area; avoid fast pumping motions of the arms
Bursitis— Inflammation of fluid-filled sacs located near knees, hips, shoulders, or elbows	Pain and stiffness in the area of the bursa; pain is the same at rest or with movement	Direct pressure or overuse of muscles in the area of the bursa; muscle imbalance, improper progression of resistance or impact activities	Proper alignment and proper strength-training techniques; add resistance gradually ℞: If swelling or reduced motion is present, ice the area and limit exercise until symptoms subside

TABLE 5-1—cont'd
Overuse Injuries, Conditions, Symptoms, Causes, Prevention and Treatment

Injury	Symptoms	Possible cause	Prevention/Medical treatment (℞)
Forefoot pain (metatarsalgia)— Bruising of the metatarsal heads	General pain in the ball of the foot, particularly at the base of the 2nd and 3rd toes	Repeated high impact forces to the ball of the foot; insufficient forefoot cushioning; activities such as dancing in high heels	Wear shoes with adequate cushioning and support; substitute low impact or nonimpact activities ℞: Ice; rest
Iliotibial band syndrome— Irritation of the connective tissue band along the outer thigh	Tenderness on the outside of the knee	Overuse, poor mechanics and alignment of the knees; muscular imbalance	Gentle daily stretching of the IT band; proper alignment and movement execution ℞: Ice; rest; modify mechanics
Lower back pain— Mechanical stress to various muscles, ligaments, joints, or nerves of the lower back	Pain, tenderness to touch, swelling, stiffness, loss of motion, or referred pain to the legs	Poor posture, poor body mechanics and exercise technique; lack of pelvic stabilization	Adequate strength and flexibility; pelvic stabilization; good postural habits and proper mechanics of lifting; avoid fast or flexed and twisting movements of the back such as opposite toe touches ℞: Ice, rest, mild stretches, consult a medical professional
Muscle strain— Overstretching or tearing of muscle tissue or tendon	Localized tenderness and swelling	Inadequate warm-up; inflexibility of muscle; muscle imbalance around a joint; ballistic stretching with inadequate warm-up	Adequate warm-up; balanced stretching and strength development of muscles around each joint ℞: Ice, mild stretching, modify activities

Continued

TABLE 5-1—cont'd
Overuse Injuries, Conditions, Symptoms, Causes, Prevention and Treatment

Injury	Symptoms	Possible cause	Prevention/Medical treatment (R)
Neuroma (forefoot pain)— Pinching of a nerve between the third and fourth toes	Swelling and sharp pain radiating to the ends of the toes	Repeated impact to the ball of the foot; inadequate cushioning of the forefoot; shoes that are too narrow	Proper sizing and forefoot support in shoes R: Ice, avoid impact activities; consult a medical professional
Patellofemoral syndrome (knee pain)— Improper tracking of the kneecap in the groove of the femur may result in damage to the cartilage behind the kneecap	Pain with ascending or descending stairs; possible grinding, clicking or grating around the knee joint	Various causes: poor mechanics, poor alignment of kneecap or feet; excessive knee flexion and extension against heavy resistance	Vary impact; wear supportive shoes with good arch support and cushioning; avoid activities that cause pain R: Consult a medical professional regarding possible muscle imbalances and alignment correction
Plantar fasciitis— Inflammation of the connective tissue of the foot, particularly at the instep	Extreme tenderness of the instep in the morning, decreasing throughout the day; pain may radiate along the arch of the foot	High arch of the foot with inadequate support; repeated high impact activities; inadequate ankle flexibility	Flexible shoes with adequate arch support; limiting high impact activities on nonresilient surfaces; regular stretching of the calf R: Ice; seek medical attention if pain persists
Rotator cuff injury— Strain, impingement or irritation to the tendons of the rotators of the shoulder	Shoulder pain with possible decrease in range of motion forceful twisting or a fall on an outstretched arm	Overuse, improper mechanics of throwing or weight-lifting; of rotators and shoulder girdle muscles, adequate warm-up	Balanced stretching of the rotators, gradual strengthening R: Ice for pain relief; seek medical attention for persistent pain

TABLE 5-1—cont'd
Overuse Injuries, Conditions, Symptoms, Causes, Prevention and Treatment

Injury	Symptoms	Possible cause	Prevention/Medical treatment (℞)
Shin splints— Various conditions resulting in pain of the lower leg	Pain, tenderness to palpation, possible swelling of the front or side of the lower leg	Improper progression of impact activities; inadequate warm-up; changing surfaces; inadequate shoe support	Vary impact, gradually increase intensity, frequency, and duration of exercises; thorough warm-up; adequate shoes ℞: Ice for pain relief; limit impact activities
Shoulder impingement— Compression of the front or side structures of the shoulder joint	Pain over the affected areas of the shoulder	Muscle imbalance of the shoulder and shoulder girdle; poor alignment of the upper torso during shoulder motion	Balance strength and flexibility of the shoulder, chest, and upper back muscles; use proper weight-training technique and progression
Stress fractures— Bone breakdown in an area of excessive stress (usually foot or shin)	Specific, sharp pain with tenderness to touch directly over the affected bone, increasing with impact	Improper progression of exercise intensity; improper footwear on unyielding surfaces	Adequate warm-up and progression of exercise intensity; supportive footwear; vary impact bearing activities; ℞: Substitute non-weight activities; ice for pain relief

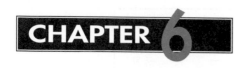

CHAPTER 6

YOUR ACTION PLAN:
EXERCISE
AND BODY COMPOSITION

OBJECTIVES

After reading this chapter, you should be able to do the following:

- Understand that your optimal weight may be very different from what a standard height and weight chart, societal pressure, or peer values seem to dictate.
- Discuss the differences between various methods for measuring body composition.
- Outline a plan of action for safely and effectively altering body composition.
- Understand the role of heredity in certain predetermined factors that influence how much, where, and when your body stores fat.
- Establish the link between sound dietary change and a healthy lifestyle.

KEY TERMS

While reading this chapter, you will become familiar with the following terms:

- ▶ **Essential Body Fat**
- ▶ **Genetics**
- ▶ **Overfat**
- ▶ **Overweight**

UNDERSTANDING BODY COMPOSITION

Chapter 2 identified body composition as one of the key components of fitness, defining it as the division of your total body weight into two components: fat weight and lean weight (muscle, bones, internal organs). If body composition is so much more important than weight, then why can everyone tell you what they weigh (and what they think they should weigh)? Why does virtually every household in America have at least one scale even though most people have never had their body fat measured? It is interesting that what many persons think they *should* weigh is often based on factors that are difficult to quantify, such as societal pressure, peer values, and misperceptions of body type. Most people use a scale to measure body weight because it is fast, easy, and inexpensive. What they do not know is that scale weight does not give worthwhile information because it cannot distinguish between fat and lean weight.

In the past, insurance and other industries have used normative charts to predict what someone supposedly should weigh based on height and used those values to establish insurance risk. Your *optimal weight*, however, may be very different from what a standard height/weight chart would predict—especially if you are a lean exerciser. Can you be **overfat** without being **overweight**? You bet! To help you see this, compare Sarah Sedentary and Annie Active, who are both 5 feet 6 inches tall with "large" frames (Figure 6-1). According to the height/weight charts Sarah weighs just what she should at 140 pounds, but she has 29% body fat. This means that Sarah has 41 pounds of fat and 99 pounds of lean weight. Annie, who weighs 150 pounds, is "overweight," but she has only 20% body fat. Annie has only 30 pounds of fat and 120 pounds of lean weight. Annie is over*weight* according to the height/weight charts, but she is certainly not over*fat*. Sarah, on the other hand, is at her ideal weight according to the height/weight charts, but she is over*fat*. Your body fat, rather than your body weight or frame size, should be the criterion for determining whether you are fit or fat and maintaining a healthy body weight.

So what should your body fat be? Most experts recommend that men be between 15% and 20% fat and women between 20% and 26%. Why the difference between men and women? Women have more **essential body fat** than men. Up to 12% of a woman's body fat can be essential fat, or fat the body stores to be able to perform necessary metabolic functions. For women, those functions tend to

▶ **Overfat**
Having a higher percentage of body fat than what is considered healthy, which could put you at risk for certain health problems.

▶ **Overweight**
An ambiguous term that does not accurately assess whether someone is at higher risk for certain health problems.

▶ **Essential Body Fat**
Fat the body stores to be able to perform necessary metabolic functions (up to about 12% for women and 3% for men).

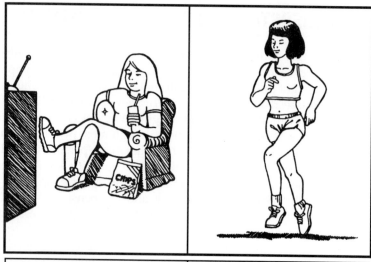

Sarah Sedentary	Annie Active
140 lb	150 lb
29% fat	20% fat
41 lb fat	30 lb fat
99 lb lean	120 lb lean

FIGURE 6-1 Sarah Sedentary and Annie Active.

be related to hormones and the ability to become pregnant. Men, on the average, have a much lower essential body fat of about 3%.

MEASURING BODY COMPOSITION

How do you find out how much lean and fat weight you have? A number of different methods can be used to determine body composition. One of them is hydrostatic, or underwater, weighing. Considered the best means of body composition assessment, underwater weighing works on the basic principle that fat (which is less dense than muscle) will float and muscle will sink in water. Thus someone with a high percentage of body fat will weigh less under water when compared with a leaner person. Most research studies use underwater weighing because of its accuracy. The potential drawbacks are that it requires expensive equipment and that it is not very user friendly. It relies on the subject to be totally submerged, fully exhale, and remain still enough to establish an underwater scale weight.

Skinfold measurements (Figure 6-2) are another common form of body composition assessment, which are more cost effective and less difficult for most persons. The tester simply measures the thickness of fat directly beneath the skin in a number of areas to predict body fat based on the sum of the skinfolds and the age of the person. Skinfolds can be quite accurate, although they may overestimate or underestimate percent of body fat on certain persons who tend to have body fat in different areas or who carry fat more internally rather than at the surface.

Bioelectrical impedance is a fairly new technique for determining body composition. Impedance works by passing a small electrical current between two electrodes. Because fat-free mass contains most of the water and conducting electrolytes in the body, the electrical current moves quickly through muscle, while fat impedes the current. The overall accuracy of impedance is similar to that of skinfolds, but it overestimates body fat in lean persons and underestimates it in fatter persons.

Bear in mind that accuracy rates for all the methods can vary significantly depending on the technique used and the training of the tester. The Kellogg's pinch an inch test (Figure 6-3), where you see if you can pinch a thickness of more than an inch at the back of the arm or abdominal area, is a less scientific but visually reliable indicator of whether or not you have excess body fat.

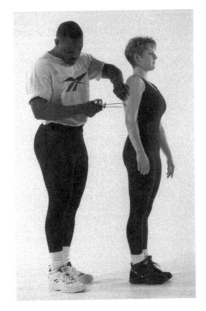

FIGURE 6-2   Skinfold measurements.

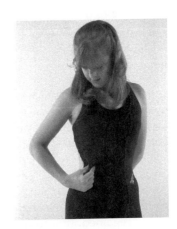

FIGURE 6-3   Kellogg's pinch an inch test.

ALTERING BODY COMPOSITION

So what if you are overfat? Well, first of all, being overfat is directly or indirectly associated with diseases that account for 15% to 20% of the annual U.S. mortality. These include coronary artery disease, high blood pressure, diabetes, elevated triglycerides and total cholesterol, thromboembolic disease, congestive heart failure, and increased risk during surgery. It is estimated that the average American will gain about a pound of fat each year after the age of 25 and will lose about one-half pound of muscle and bone each year. This change would represent a 30-pound fat gain between the ages of 25 and 55! *Now* is the time to establish and maintain a desirable body composition.

What can you do about a high body fat percentage? Your options are pretty basic:

- Diet by reducing caloric intake
- Exercise
- Combine diet with exercise

DIET OR EXERCISE, ALONE, IS NOT ENOUGH

As mentioned earlier, a well balanced, nutrient-dense diet combined with regular aerobic exercise is the best way to lose fat and maintain lean muscle mass. First we will consider diet and exercise separately, and then see how the combination can be more effective than either diet or exercise alone.

▶ Diet Alone

Many persons prefer dieting to lose weight, thinking that weight loss is just a matter of willpower. The ACSM states that diet only as a means of weight loss usually results in moderate losses of water and lean body mass in addition to fat. Dieting also seems to be associated with a reduction in basal metabolic rate. This is especially true with very low calorie diets (less than 1000 calories per day). Such a low caloric intake is not able to supply all the essential nutrients and will generally lead to a reduction in metabolism. When you go off the diet, caloric intake returns to normal, but the metabolism might not, leading to further weight gain.

Some persons use high protein, low carbohydrate diets simply because the scale appears to show substantial weight loss each week. Remember, though, that your scale cannot show what kind of weight you lost! Because you store large quantities of water along with carbohydrate, when you cut out the carbohydrate, you also cut out the water storage. Thus the majority of weight apparently lost with this type of low calorie diet is attributed to water loss rather than fat loss and is quickly regained. In addition, high protein diets can be potentially damaging to the liver and kidneys and negatively affect other bodily functions. You can safely lose only about 2 pounds of fat each week; losses any greater than that are usually from water or muscle mass or both. The Fitness Tip on the following page gives the very simple options available for healthy weight loss.

Because the ACSM indicates that the major objective of any weight-reduction program should be to lose body fat while maintaining lean body mass, diet alone is not recommended as an effective plan. In fact, reducing caloric intake only moderately (500 calories below baseline intake) without adding exercise into the picture will lead to a loss of water and lean tissue, rather than of mainly fat weight.

Fitness Tip

Options for Weight Loss

1. Diet: reduced metabolism; water and lean loss

2. Exercise: slow but effective

3. Diet + Exercise: best method; decrease caloric intake, increase caloric expenditure

▶ Exercise Alone

How does exercise affect weight loss? Exercise alone as a means of weight loss can be effective, but expect it to be a slow and steady loss. One pound of fat contains about 3500 calories, and it would take a lot of exercise to use that much energy! Studies indicate that there are slight decreases in total body weight and fat weight and increases in lean weight with exercise. The most important factor in exercise and weight control or loss is *the total number of calories expended*. If two workouts have about the same caloric expenditure, you will see about the same results in weight maintenance or loss.

To promote weight loss, exercise programs should be designed to burn more calories. Increasing frequency and duration with a low exercise intensity is really the best way to do this. If weight loss (fat reduction) is an exercise goal, a guideline to consider is the ACSM recommendation that you expend at least *300 Calories per session if you work out three times a week; 200 Calories per session four times a week*. A 132-pound woman, for example, would expend 300 Calories with the following activities:

- Step aerobics (8-inch step) = 32 minutes
- Running = 3 miles
- Walking = 4.7 miles
- High intensity aerobics = 30 minutes
- Jazzercise/step = 35 minutes

See Chapter 12 for additional information that will help you determine your approximate caloric expenditure for aerobic dance as well as other activities.

DIET + EXERCISE = THE IDEAL COMBINATION

The best weight loss program combines balanced nutrition with exercise. Although most persons are looking for a "quick fix" it helps to understand that weight that is lost quickly is usually quickly regained. Stringent diets that remove food entirely by substituting shakes or drinks do little to help you learn how to make wise food choices.

How do you know what are safe and effective changes to make if you're interested in decreasing body fat? The ACSM summarizes the traits of a desirable weight loss program as follows:

1. Eat at least 1200 Calories per day. Going below 1200 Calories may affect your metabolic rate and will not allow you to eat a nutritionally complete diet.
2. Choose and adapt foods that you like, that are easy to find and prepare and that fit in your budget.
3. Because gradual weight loss is safer and less likely to affect your metabolism, weight loss should be no more than 2.2 pounds each week. Reduce your caloric intake by no more than 500 to 1000 Calories per day.
4. Determine *why* you eat, not just *what* you eat. Identify eating habits and patterns that trigger unhealthy eating patterns and look for ways to make changes. For example, if you snack on fatty foods while you study, do not stop studying! Substitute some low fat alternatives (pretzels, sorbet, etc.), study in a location that does not allow food, or take frequent exercise breaks to get up and moving.
5. Combine an aerobic exercise program with any reduction in caloric intake. The added exercise may help offset the reduction in metabolism caused by cutting calories and should also help you feel better and increase your energy levels.
6. Do not go "on" a diet because that implies you will at some point go "off" the diet! Make changes in your eating and exercise habits that you can maintain for a lifetime. Think of making lifestyle changes rather than looking for a short-term temporary solution that has short-term, temporary results. The Fitness Tip below provides a summary of information for a desirable weight-loss program.

Fitness Tip

Desirable Weight–Loss Program

1. 1200 Calories a day.
2. Reasonable foods.
3. Lose no more than 2.2 pounds a week; reduce caloric intake no more than 500 to 1000 Calories a day.
4. Evaluate *why* you eat; make changes.
5. Combine caloric reduction with increased activity levels.
6. Make lifestyle changes.

THE ROLE OF HEREDITY

All of the preceding information does not, however, work out like the simple mathematical formula of a + b = c, or diet + exercise = your image of a perfect body. A sound diet and regular exercise are part of a healthy lifestyle, but your **genetics** also play an important role in the area of body composition. Most obviously, your genetic makeup determined whether you were going to be male or female. You were fashioned from an entirely unique genetic code that dictated everything from the color of your hair to when your first teeth would appear to the length and shape of your nose! How your genetics affect your body composition becomes more evident as you grow and develop. You have no control, for example, over how many and what type of fat cells you will be born with (we all have millions!) or where the fat cells will be deposited (usually not where you would choose for them to be!).

What you *want* to see happen as you develop a healthy lifestyle and what *can* happen based on your genetics may be two very different things. Many women, for example, would like to change the shape of their hip and thigh area and often spend years dieting and exercising while appearing to accomplish very little. What's the problem? Fat tends to be deposited in these areas on most women in response to estrogen production and another hormone called lipoprotein lipase. The activity of this hormone is particularly high in the hip and thigh region of women, while fat mobilization from this area is low. This hormonal interaction leads to increased fat deposits, and the whole cycle appears to be linked with reproduction. So, although diet and exercise can have some impact, recognize that they cannot negate other physiologic mechanisms in the process.

SOUND DIETARY CHANGE

What dietary changes should you make if you decide to reduce caloric intake? The best intervention appears to be reducing fat in your diet while at the same time looking at total caloric intake. When you evaluated your fat intake and established goals for change in Chapter 4 you should have seen that a fat intake of 25% or less is ideal. Although this may not be realistic for all persons, watching the amount of fat in your diet should be the focus of any changes you make, particularly if your fat intake is over 40%.

Only counting fat grams, though, does not give you the complete picture. Many "light," "low-fat" or even "fat-free" foods have little to no fat but are

▶ **Genetics**
Play a major role in body composition and sometimes are a limiting factor, in that one cannot negate physiologic mechanisms such as how many or what type of fat cells you were born with or where the fat cells will be deposited.

very high in total calories and loaded with sugar. Your best bet is to follow the new inverted pyramid food guide. This new structure reflects the emphasis on complex carbohydrates (fruits, vegetables, grains, pasta, potatoes) with fewer calories coming from protein, fat, and foods high in simple sugars. Chapter 7 has additional nutritional and dietary information to help you develop a healthy eating plan.

The goal of any weight-loss program should be greater than simply losing weight. This is your chance to begin to develop eating and exercise habits that you can continue forever. At the same time, you can begin to establish healthy lifestyle expectations that reflect a balanced perspective of total body fitness. The most effective means to lose weight is a combination of diet and exercise: the most effective way to keep it off is to maintain the healthy habits that helped you achieve your goal.

SUMMARY

- Traditional height/weight charts don't take body composition into account: you can be overfat without being overweight.
- Everyone needs a certain amount of essential body fat to maintain necessary metabolic functions.
- A combination of appropriate dietary changes and increased exercise will ensure that one is losing fat as opposed to lean or water weight.
- If you want to lose weight make sure you eat at least 1200 Calories a day, select foods that are easy to find and prepare, lose no more than 2.2 pounds a week, evaluate why you eat, combine calorie reduction with increased levels of physical activity and make lifestyle changes that will become a part of your routine for years to come.
- Low-fat foods are not necessarily low in calories. If you are monitoring your diet, be sure to read the nutritional labels on foods to pick foods that are low in calories and fat.

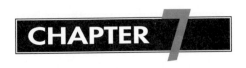

CHAPTER 7

OBJECTIVES

After reading this chapter, you should be able to do the following:

- Discuss the basic concepts of balanced nutrition.
- Consider a system of food choices that provides a well-selected variety of foods.
- Understand how to use the food guide pyramid to choose a variety of foods that meet your daily nutritional requirements.
- Read food labels to determine what is actually considered a serving and identify the percentage of fat per serving.

KEY TERMS

While reading this chapter, you will become familiar with the following terms:

- ▶ Carbohydrates
- ▶ Macronutrients
- ▶ Nutrient-dense
- ▶ Nutrients
- ▶ Serving

BASE OF KNOWLEDGE

The arena of nutrition research is a relatively new one in the scientific field, beginning in the early 1900s with the discovery of vitamins. Every year and a half, continuing research doubles the amount of nutrition information available. It is sometimes difficult to distinguish hype and misconceptions from fact, but the old saying "you are what you eat" is continually reinforced by available studies.

As you make a concerted effort to improve health, appearance, body composition, and athletic performance, making the effort to learn sound nutritional information is particularly important. Do not fall for dietary regimens that contribute nothing and may even be harmful to your overall health and fitness.

SEPARATING FACT FROM FICTION

The Food and Nutrition Science Alliance (FANSA) has published several recommendations that may help as you learn how to evaluate new information about nutrition. FANSA represents over 100,000 experts in the fields of medicine, nutrition, and food science. They suggest that you be wary of claims that seem too good to be true or promise a quick fix, or that are refuted by reputable scientific organizations. Many claims are supported by "studies," but recommendations should not be based on a single study, on studies without peer review, or on overly simplified conclusions from a complex study. Also beware of lists of "good" or "bad" foods or dire warnings about a single product or regimen.

BASICS OF NUTRITION

The basic components of food are called **nutrients**. Nutrients supply the body's need for energy, growth, and repair and help to regulate the chemical reactions and mechanisms of the body. The six categories of nutrients include water, carbohydrates, proteins, fats, vitamins, and minerals.

Earlier in this book, we addressed the importance of adequate water consumption for exercise. Water is essential for temperature control and effective transportation of nutrients to and waste from exercising muscles. Water is also important in energy production and other essential chemical reactions in the body. Most experts recommend drinking at least eight glasses of water per day. Any beverage can contribute to this amount except those containing caffeine or alcohol, which tend to dehydrate rather than hydrate.

Carbohydrates, proteins, and fats are known as **macronutrients.** They are consumed in relatively large amounts (compared to vitamins and minerals) and are the source of the body's energy. The calories and chemical components supplied by these nutrients build and repair tissue and fuel the processes that occur constantly to sustain life.

Quantities of energy supplied by food are referred to as kilocalories or Calories (with a capital C). Carbohydrates and proteins supply 4 Calories per gram and fat supplies 9 Calories per gram. Stated in more familiar terms, proteins and carbohydrates contain 112 Calories per ounce, and an ounce of fat has 252 Calories. Alcohol, though not a food, also contains calories. Alcohol has 7 Calories per gram (196 Calories per ounce), almost as much as fat. Calories consumed in excess of the body's current need for energy are converted and stored as fat.

CARBOHYDRATES

Carbohydrates are classified as either simple or complex, although they both supply the same amount of energy (4 Cal/gm). Simple carbohydrates occur naturally along with vitamins and minerals in fruits and milk. Refined sugars such as corn syrup, honey, and table sugar are also sources of simple carbohydrates, but without additional nutrients: they are often referred to as "empty calories."

Complex carbohydrates are more complicated chains of sugars or starches that are found in vegetables, fruits, whole grains, cereals, and dried peas and beans. They also occur naturally in combination with vitamins, minerals, and fiber. The current U.S. dietary guidelines recommend that over half (about 58%) of your calories be supplied by carbohydrates, particularly complex carbohydrates (because of the associated vitamins, minerals, and fiber). They recommend that refined sugars be limited to 10% of your calories. For example, in an eating plan of 2000 Calories, approximately 1160 Calories should come from carbohydrates, with no more than 200 Calories from refined sugars.

Carbohydrates break down to glucose (also known as blood sugar) during digestion and are absorbed by the bloodstream to supply the energy needs of the brain and nervous system. Glucose is also recombined by the body and stored in muscle tissue and the liver as glycogen. Glycogen is the first, most readily available fuel supply for aerobic activities.

PROTEINS

Proteins also supply energy (4 Cal/gm). They are composed of amino acids, the "building blocks" of all body tissue, hormones, and enzymes. Dietary sources of protein include meat, milk, fish, poultry, cheese, tofu, and eggs. The full spectrum of amino acids is also present in certain combinations of grains and vegetables (such as pasta primavera or beans and rice) or grains with milk products (such as cereal and milk).

▶ **Nutrients**
Basic components of food that supply the body's need for energy, growth, and repair and help to regulate the chemical reactions and mechanisms of the body.

▶ **Macronutrients**
Carbohydrates, proteins, and fats, which are the source of the body's energy for building and repairing tissue and fueling the processes needed to sustain life.

Current U.S. dietary guidelines recommend that only 12% of your calories come from protein. So in an eating plan of 2000 Calories, only 240 should come from protein. Most Americans consume excess protein, which is then converted and stored as fat. Even with high powered strength training, it is likely that a person would be able to get sufficient protein from his or her food without additional protein supplementation. Too much protein in the diet can also be harmful, leading to kidney damage or other medical problems.

FATS

Fat supplies essential fatty acids, and plays a role in the insulation and protection of organs and in the absorption of certain vitamins. Current guidelines recommend that no more than 30% of your daily Calories come from fat. For example, in an eating plan of 2000 Calories, only 600 Calories should come from fat. Several health organizations recommend lower percentages to prevent specific diseases. The average American diet, however, is closer to 40% fat. Excess fat consumption not only is stored as fat, causing obesity, but also contributes to diseases, such as high blood pressure and diabetes.

Excess fat consumption may be related to several factors. Fat is a hidden component of many foods, it tastes good to the American palate, and it has a certain satiety factor. That is, fat makes you feel satisfied or full because it stays in your stomach longer for digestion.

▶ Consumption of Fat and Body Composition

One of the keys to controlling body composition through a sound eating plan is to eat enough calories; avoid crash diets that lower the metabolic rate. Make sure the calories you consume are "**nutrient-dense**" by limiting the empty calories (refined sugars, fat, and alcohol). Spend your calorie budget on the calories that are dense with additional nutrients that supply vitamins, minerals, fiber, amino acids, and the essential fatty acids. Refer to your BMR calculation in Chapter 3 to get an idea of your basal caloric needs. Sample diets of 1600, 2200, and 2800 Calories are provided in Table 7-1. Remember to increase your caloric intake for additional physical activity as well as for structured workouts.

VITAMINS

Vitamins are necessary in small amounts to regulate the chemical reactions of the body. Vitamins themselves provide no calories, and therefore provide no energy. Each of the thirteen vitamins serves a special function and must be obtained from the diet. The U.S. Department of Agriculture (USDA) recommends consuming certain amounts of each vitamin daily through a variety of foods. Most experts agree that it may be difficult to obtain the recommended amounts if you are consuming less than 1600 to 1800 total Calories a day. If that is the case,

TABLE 7-1
Sample Diets for a Day at Three Caloric Levels

	Low (about 1600)*	Moderate (about 2200)†	High (about 2800)‡
Bread Group Servings	6	6	11
Vegetable Group Servings	3	4	5
Fruit Group Servings	2	3	4
Milk Group Servings	2-3§	2-3§	2-3§
Meat Group Servings† (ounces)	5	6	7
Total Fat‡ (grams)	53	73	93
Total Added Sugars§ (tsp)	6	12	18

From How to make the pyramid work for you, Washington, DC, 1995, US Department of Agriculture and US Department of Health and Human Services.
*1600 calories is about right for many sedentary women and some older adults
†2200 calories is about right for most children, teenage girls, active women, and many sedentary men. Women who are pregnant or breast-feeding may need somewhat more.
‡2800 calories is about right for teenage boys, many active men, and some very active women.
§Women who are pregnant or breast-feeding, teenagers, and young adults to age 24 need 3 servings.

you might want to check with a nutritionist to see if vitamin supplementation is appropriate.

MINERALS

Like vitamins, minerals are essential for health. They are involved in a variety of internal functions, such as forming insulin (zinc), hemoglobin (iron), bones and teeth (calcium, phosphorus), and regulating heart rhythm and muscle contraction (calcium, sodium, potassium). Like vitamins, minerals must be obtained from the diet. They must also be properly balanced for optimal absorption and utilization.

GUIDELINES FOR BALANCED NUTRITION

Over 40 nutrients are considered to be essential by most experts. The Recommended Daily Allowances (RDAs) as defined by the National Research Council of the National Academy of Sciences contain the amounts of these nutrients needed daily to maintain health (Table 7-2).

▶ **Nutrient-dense**
Foods that are nutrient-dense contribute more to the nutrient needs of your body than to the energy needs.

Category	Age (years) or Condition	Weight[b] (kg)	(lb)	Height[b] (cm)	(in)	Protein (g)	Fat-Soluble Vitamins Vitamin A (µg RE)[c]	Vitamin D (µg)[d]	Vitamin E (mg α-TE)[e]	Vitamin K (µg)	Water-Soluble Vitamins Vitamin C (mg)	Thiamin (mg)	Riboflavin (mg)	Niacin (mg NE)[f]	Vitamin B$_6$ (mg)	Folate (µg)	Vitamin B$_{12}$ (µg)	Minerals Calcium (mg)	Phosphorus (mg)	Magnesium (mg)	Iron (mg)	Zinc (mg)	Iodine (µg)	Selenium (µg)
Males	15-18	66	145	176	69	59	1000	10	10	65	60	1.5	1.8	20	2.0	200	2.0	1200	1200	400	12	15	150	50
	19-24	72	160	177	70	58	1000	10	10	70	60	1.5	1.7	19	2.0	200	2.0	1200	1200	350	10	15	150	70
	25-50	79	174	176	70	63	1000	5	10	80	60	1.5	1.7	19	2.0	200	2.0	800	800	350	10	15	150	70
	51+	77	170	173	68	63	1000	5	10	80	60	1.2	1.4	15	2.0	200	2.0	800	800	350	10	15	150	70
Females	15-18	55	120	163	64	44	800	10	8	55	60	1.1	1.3	15	1.5	180	2.0	1200	1200	300	15	12	150	50
	19-24	58	128	164	65	46	800	10	8	60	60	1.1	1.3	15	1.6	180	2.0	1200	1200	280	15	12	150	55
	25-50	63	138	163	64	50	800	5	8	65	60	1.1	1.3	15	1.6	180	2.0	800	800	280	15	12	150	55
	51+	65	143	160	63	50	800	5	8	65	60	1.0	1.2	13	1.6	180	2.0	800	800	280	10	12	150	55
Pregnant						60	800	10	10	65	70	1.5	1.6	17	2.2	400	2.2	1200	1200	320	30	15	175	65
Lactating	1st 6 months					65	1300	10	12	65	95	1.6	1.8	20	2.1	280	2.6	1200	1200	355	15	19	200	75
	2nd 6 months					62	1200	10	11	65	90	1.6	1.7	20	2.1	260	2.6	1200	1200	340	15	16	200	75

Reprinted with permission from Recommended Dietary Allowances, ed 10, Copyright © 1989, National Academy Press, Washington D.C.

[a]The allowances, expressed as average daily intakes over time, are intended to provide for individual variations among most normal persons, since they live in the United States under usual environmental stresses. Diets should be based on a variety of common foods to provide other nutrients for which human requirements have been less well defined. See text for detailed discussion of allowances and of nutrients not tabulated.

[b]Weights and heights of reference adults are actual median for the U.S. population of the designated age, as reported by NHANES II. The use of these figures does not imply that the weight-to-height ratios are ideal.

[c]Retinol equivalents. 1 retinol equivalent = 1 µg retinol or 6 µg β-carotene.

[d]As cholecalciferol. 10 µg cholecalciferol = 400 IU of Vitamin D.

[e]α-Tocopherol equivalents. 1 mg d-α tocopherol = 1 α-TE.

[f]1 NE (niacin equivalent) is equal to 1 mg of niacin or 60 mg of dietary tryptophan.

The Dietary Guidelines for Americans is also a set of recommendations that relate to percentages of carbohydrate, protein, and fat in the daily diet, as described previously in this chapter. They have been accepted by many health organizations in the United States, not only in the promotion of optimal health but also in the prevention of diseases such as cancer, diabetes, cardiovascular disease, and high blood pressure. These guidelines recommend decreased consumption of high-fat foods (oils, margarine, fatty meats, and whole dairy products), cholesterol rich foods (eggs and organ meats), refined sugars, salt, and processed foods. They recommend increased consumption of fresh vegetables and fruits, whole grain cereals and bread, and dried beans and peas and limited meat consumption through substitution with fish, plant proteins, and poultry.

In order for these recommendations to be practical, you must be able to translate the percentages of carbohydrate, protein, and fat in the daily diet into "How much of which foods should I eat?" The Food Guide Pyramid from the U.S. Department of Health and Human Services (DHHS) (Figure 7-1) provides a way to do this. It is designed to help with food choices and meal-planning and to develop a balanced nutritional program that contains adequate and appropriate nutrients and calories. It gives the number of servings of each type of food that the general population should consume.

HOW MUCH IS A SERVING?

The next step for applying this information in a practical way is to know how much food is considered to be a **serving**. Servings within a food group deliver equivalent amounts of nutrients, but the calorie content may vary widely, depending on the fat content and method of preparation. For example, one serving of milk equals 8 ounces of low-fat milk or 1⅓ cups of vanilla ice cream. These two items provide equivalent nutrients, but the low-fat milk contains 102 Calories while the vanilla ice cream contains 353 Calories! The Fitness Tip on page 115 defines a serving as determined by the USDA and the DHHS.

To bridge the gap between what constitutes a serving on paper and what you find as you sit down to eat, let's take a closer look. In the meat group one serving is 3 ounces of meat (roughly the size of the meat patty in a Big Mac hamburger). Do not fool yourself into thinking that one piece of meat is just one serving: a 12-ounce steak, after cooking, is approximately 3.5 servings. Instead, mentally picture that Big Mac hamburger and compare the size with what is on your plate.

Text continued on p. 116

▶ **Serving**
Determined amount of foods within a food group that delivers equivalent amounts of nutrients. It is important to note that calorie content of a serving within a food group can vary depending on fat content and method of preparation of a particular food.

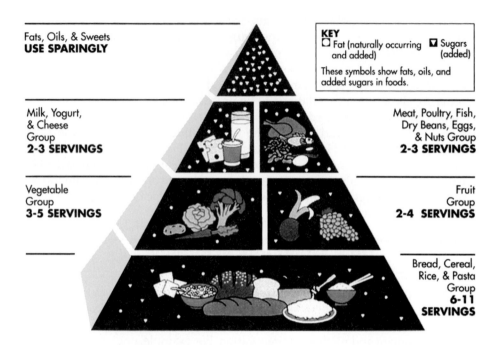

FIGURE 7-1 USDA's Food Guide Pyramid. Choose foods from each of the five food groups. The Food Guide Pyramid illustrates the importance of balance among food groups in a daily eating pattern. Most of the daily servings of food should be selected from the food groups that are the largest in the picture and closest to the base of the Pyramid.

- Choose most of your foods from the grain products group (6 to 11 servings), the vegetable group (3 to 5 servings), and the fruit group (2 to 4 servings).
- Eat moderate amounts of foods from the milk group (2 to 3 servings) and the meat and beans group (2 to 3 servings).
- Choose sparingly foods that provide few nutrients and are high in fat and sugars.

NOTE: A range of servings is given for each food group. The smaller number is for people who consume about 1600 Calories a day and are sedentary. The larger number is for those who consume about 2800 Calories a day and are more active.

From US Department of Agriculture and US Department of Health and Human Services: Nutrition and your health: dietary guidelines for Americans, ed.4, Washington DC, 1995.

Fitness Tip

What Counts as a Serving?*

Grain Products Group (bread, cereal, rice, and pasta)

1 slice of bread
1 ounce of ready-to-eat cereal
½ cup of cooked cereal, rice, or pasta

Vegetable Group

1 cup of raw leafy vegetables
½ cup of other vegetables—cooked or chopped raw
¾ cup of vegetable juice

Fruit Group

1 medium apple, banana, orange
½ cup of chopped, cooked, or canned fruit
¾ cup of fruit juice

Milk Group (milk, yogurt, and cheese)

1 cup of milk or yogurt
1½ ounces of natural cheese
2 ounces of processed cheese

Meat and Beans Group (meat, poultry, fish, dry beans, eggs, and nuts)

2 to 3 ounces of cooked lean meat, poultry, or fish
½ cup of cooked dry beans or 1 egg counts as 1 ounce of lean meat. Two tablespoons of peanut butter or ⅓ cup of nuts count as 1 ounce of meat.

*Some foods fit into more than one group. Dry beans, peas, and lentils can be counted as servings in either the beans group or vegetable group. These "cross over" foods can be counted as servings from either one or the other group, but not both. Serving sizes indicated here are those used in the Food Guide Pyramid and based on both suggested and usually consumed portions necessary to achieve adequate nutrient intake. They differ from serving sizes on the Nutrition Facts Label, which reflect portions usually consumed.
From US Department of Agriculture and US Department of Health and Human Services: Nutrition and your health: dietary guidelines for Americans, ed. 4, Washington DC, 1995.

One serving of fish is 4.5 ounces, providing the same nutrients (but less fat) as 3.5 ounces of meat. For the nonanimal protein sources such as beans and legumes (low fat) or nuts and seeds (high fat) one meat serving is 1 cup.

In the milk group, the serving size of liquids is 8 ounces. As the water content decreases in other milk-group foods, the size of the serving decreases: one serving of yogurt is ⅔ cup, cottage cheese is ½ cup, hard cheese is 1½ ounces (a little more than one of those prewrapped cheese slices). As mentioned earlier, a serving size of ice cream is 1⅓ cups. Good news? Hardly. Ice cream has such poor nutrient value that it takes that much to supply enough nutrients for a serving. The Calorie content is also exponentially higher! For example, the Calories in one serving of low-fat milk (1% fat) is 102, in whole yogurt, 227, and vanilla ice cream, 353.

The standard serving size of fruits and vegetables is 1 cup. To estimate the number of servings of a whole fruit or vegetable, mentally chop it up and put in a 1-cup measure. For juice or dried fruit the serving size is ½ cup, but the sugar content increases dramatically here.

In breads and cereals, the standard serving is one slice of bread; so buns, bagels, etc. would actually be two servings. For cereals and grains, the serving size is 1 ounce of cooked food such as rice, barley, or corn. Cereals vary according to their density. For example, one serving of Grape-Nuts is ¼ cup, while one serving of flakes is ½ cup, and one serving of a "puffy" cereal like Rice Crispies is 1 cup. The chart on the side panel of a cereal box will tell you the reference serving size.

DESIGN YOUR NUTRITIONAL PLAN

Now that you have seen the Food Pyramid Guide and understand serving sizes, it is time to design your own nutritional program. Refer to your RMR calculation in Chapter 3 to get an idea of your resting Calorie needs. Add Calories to account for additional physical activity as well as structured workouts. Refer to Table 7-1 for sample nutritional programs of 1600, 2200, and 2800 Calories.

PRACTICAL WAYS TO REDUCE FAT IN YOUR DIET

As stated earlier, the average American diet is 40% fat, which is a major contributor to the increasing obesity seen in our society. Since excess dietary fat is a major problem for many, learning practical ways to reduce fat in your diet is important. The first way to get fat out of your diet is to learn to read food labels. Pay attention to the chart on the back of the package, not the big words on the front or the "natural-looking" colors or images on the label. Note the size of the serving; it may be a lot smaller than the amount you usually eat. For example, most people can eat a full bag of microwave popcorn by themselves, but some brands are **5** servings!

The next numbers of interest are the total calorie count in a serving and the fat content (grams) of each serving. To calculate the number of calories from fat, multiply the number of fat grams listed on the label by 9 (9 Calories per gram of fat). Then you can calculate the percentage of fat contained in each serving dividing the fat calories by the total calories per serving and multiplying by 100 (number of fat Calories/total Calories = % fat). Anything under 25% fat is considered "low-fat." The following box shows information from the label of a carton of sour cream.

Do not let the percentages listed on the label distract you: they are listed in terms of the percent of the recommended amount of dietary fat *if* you are consuming 2000 Calories per day. They can be very misleading if you interpret the number as the percentage of fat in that particular food. Also, do not assume that lower-fat foods are lower in calories. Many "low-fat" manufacturers add sugar to replace the flavor lost when fat is removed. The "empty" calories are the same, whether from fat or sugar! In the past few years the percentage of fat in people's diets in the United States has decreased about 3 percentage points, and the total calories consumed has increased by over 200 calories per day. Most of the unused, empty calories are stored as fat.

Fitness Tip

Nutrition Information From a Carton of Sour Cream

Serving size:	2 Tbsp (30g)
No. of servings per container:	about 8
Calories per serving:	60
Total fat:	6 g, 9%DV
Saturated fat	20%DV
Cholesterol	25 mg, 8%DV
Sodium	15 mg, 1%DV
Total carbohydrate	1 g, 0%DV
Fiber	0 g
Sugars	1 g
Protein	1 g

DV= Daily value based on a 2000 Calorie diet
Number of fat calories = 9 x 6 = 54 Calories
% fat = number of fat calories/ total calories = 54/60 = 90% fat

In addition to reading labels, you need to know how the food is prepared, making the distinction between a low-fat and high-fat preparation, such as spinach salad versus fried zucchini, or nonfat yogurt versus sour cream.

Other helpful tips include the following:

1. Limit meat consumption to 6 ounces (2 servings) daily, obtaining needed protein from beans and legumes.
2. Cut the all visible fat off meat and remove skin and fat from poultry before you cook it. Also if you roast or grill meat instead of frying and place the fat on the grill near, but not touching, the meat, you will still get some of the flavor created by the fat dripping on the coals.
3. Wean yourself from whole milk to nonfat milk products. You can accomplish this over time, giving your taste buds an opportunity to adjust, by combining whole milk with low-fat for a while, then drinking low-fat, then combine low-fat with nonfat for a while, and finally drinking nonfat alone.
4. Educate yourself about the fat content of foods at fast-food restaurants, and make selections carefully. An excellent reference for eating well when you are not cooking is *Eating on the Run* by Evelyn Tribole (Leisure Press, 1992).
5. Use "fruit-only" jams on toast and low-fat salad dressings on sandwiches instead of margarine or mayonnaise.
6. Use evaporated skim milk instead of cream for preparing sauces.
7. Look for chips that are baked, not fried, or make your own by cutting tortillas into triangles and baking at 350° F.
8. Substitute two egg whites for one whole egg.
9. Use nonfat items (nonfat cream cheese, cottage cheese, sour cream) and low-sugar desserts such as angel food cake, sorbet, and fresh fruit.

SUMMARY

- There is a vast amount of information about human nutrition, well beyond the scope of this course. Base your decisions on well documented and researched studies.
- Taking the time to investigate the subject of nutrition and preparing a healthy eating plan will not only allow you to control your body composition, but will further enhance your health.
- A nutritious diet consists of eating a variety of foods in the amounts recommended on the Food Pyramid.
- Be aware of what actually constitutes a serving in terms of prepackaged foods, and adjust your consumption accordingly.

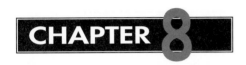

CHAPTER 8

YOUR ACTION PLAN: **CLASS COMPONENTS**

OBJECTIVES

After reading this chapter, you should be able to do the following:

- Identify the purpose and plan of execution for each of the components of a typical aerobics class.
- Use the GRACE principle for proper warm up and post aerobic cool down phases of your aerobic dance workout.
- Identify the recommended target zone of aerobic activity for each work out period.
- Evaluate the unique benefits of aerobic steady state, aerobic interval and aerobic circuit training.
- Use a variation of exercises around a muscle group to increase muscular work and progress toward overload.
- Choose the stretching technique in your cool down phase that safely increases flexibility.

KEY TERMS

While reading this chapter, you will become familiar with the following terms:

▶ Aerobic Circuit Training

▶ Aerobic Interval Training

▶ Aerobic Steady State Training

▶ Ballistic Stretching

▶ Static Stretching

CLASS FORMAT

The format for most aerobic classes is similar, beginning with a *warm-up phase* and gradually increasing intensity into the *aerobic phase* and decreasing the intensity slowly during a *post aerobic cool down. Muscular work* and a *final cool down* complete the workout. Each phase has specific purposes forming the basis for some general guidelines concerning that segment of the workout.

THE WARM-UP

Purpose. To prepare the body for the upcoming bout of exercise.

Plan. Just as you need a key to start a car engine, you need a warm-up to get your body prepared to start exercising. There are several keys to remember about the warm-up. To help remember them, think about giving yourself a GRACE period to help your body prepare for and recover from the workout. The Fitness Tip and the supporting text below provide more detail on the GRACE principle.

THINK *G*RADUAL

Movement should start slowly and build in intensity. When you increase intensity gradually, your body is able to use the warm-up period to begin some of the complex physiologic processes necessary for exercise. The term *warm-up* literally refers to an increase in tissue temperature that occurs as the body shifts blood from the core out to the working muscles in the arms and legs. It takes about 3 or 4 minutes to increase oxygen consumption and establish a new "steady state" higher than the resting level; most warm-ups will last between 5 and 10 minutes. By warming up gradually you give your body a chance to meet the increased needs of energy production and prepare the body for the remainder of the workout. One rule of thumb is that you should begin to "break a sweat" during the warm-up; it should prepare you for more vigorous exercise without wearing you out.

Fitness Tip

Warm-up Phase	
G	Gradual
R	Rehearsal
A	Action
C	Control
E	Energy

THINK *R*EHEARSAL

The warm-up is a good time to learn more difficult or complex movements that will be performed more quickly or at a higher intensity later in the workout. To obtain the maximum benefit possible during this initial phase of the workout, use it to *focus* on what you are doing and how you are doing it. Movement with control is essential, beginning with the warm-up and continuing throughout the workout.

THINK ACTION

How do you get a thick, sluggish bottle of ketchup to pour easily? You shake it up and get it moving! Even though you are not a bottle of ketchup, actively warming up decreases the thickness of the synovial fluid within the joints and enables you to move and stretch comfortably and safely. The warm-up should involve active movement before any static stretching. Most warm-ups begin with small, simple movements and progress to moves using greater muscle mass and more than one joint action. Although the possibilities are endless, some typical warm-up movements are brisk walking, step touches, and moving forward and back or side to side. The upper body should complement the lower body activity, with smooth, rhythmical movement.

THINK CONTROL

Always perform movements with control, rather than flinging or flailing. Muscular control takes practice and mental focus. Think of learning aerobics as being similar to learning how to type. Initially, you might be able to "hunt and peck" by looking at the keys while you type. It takes lots of practice (and the establishment of neuromuscular patterns) to use both hands on the keys and type without looking at the keyboard to check each individual letter. The final stage in typing—where you are thinking and typing whole words rather than letters—is difficult for most to master. You will need to establish new movement patterns if aerobic dance is a new form of exercise for you, or if your instructor consistently challenges you with new and different ways to move. Wherever you are in your movement learning curve, use the warm-up as a time to practice and establish neuromuscular control that will last throughout the workout. Rather than losing control at the end of the joint range, practice muscular control that permits you to use a full range of motion without "locking out." By controlling the muscles, you control the range of motion around a joint, which may help prevent injury.

THINK ENERGY

Do a quick mental check at the start of the workout: how are you feeling? Often your physical body reflects how you feel emotionally. That is fine if you feel super and are ready to work out; your exercise session will probably seem fun and energizing. If you are tired or wish you were somewhere else, your body tends to pick up on that and the warm-up can seem as though you are moving through mud! Try to mentally set aside this hour as a gift to yourself—and see if you do not finish feeling better about everything. Movement will affect how you feel, so pay attention to your body and focus on the positive response to your aerobics class.

THE AEROBIC PHASE

Goal for the Aerobic Phase

300 Calories per workout

Purpose. To improve aerobic fitness. For this purpose, ACSM guidelines recommend a training zone of 5 to 7 on the RPE scale (discussed in Chapter 9) and suggest that you expend at least 300 Calories per workout. This means that you will be working at what you would describe as a "somewhat hard" to "hard" pace during the aerobic portion of the workout.

Plan. There are a number of ways to exercise within the "aerobic training zone" recommended by ACSM. Three popular methods of training within these guidelines are **steady state, interval, and aerobic circuit training.**

STEADY STATE TRAINING

In steady state training, exercise intensity gradually increases to a plateau that is maintained for the duration (20+ minutes) of the aerobic segment (Figure 8-1). The plateau should represent an RPE of 5 to 7.

Unique benefit. You can sustain low- to moderate-intensity work for extended periods of time with minimal chance of injury.

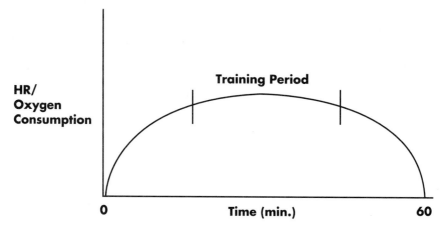

FIGURE 8-1 Aerobic steady state training.

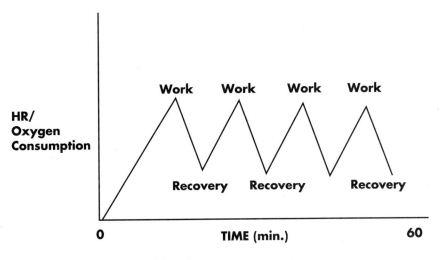

FIGURE 8-2   Aerobic interval training.

INTERVAL TRAINING

Interval segments using predominately the aerobic energy systems are generally a few minutes in length with relatively short rest periods (Figure 8-2). For example, you might work at a higher exercise intensity during a fast paced song (4 to 5 minutes) and then use a portion of the next song to keep moving at a slower pace. It is essential to listen to your body during interval training so that you minimize the risk of injury and maximize the potential benefits.

▶ **Aerobic Steady State Training**
Gradually increasing exercise intensity to a plateau that is maintained for at least 20 minutes at an RPE of 5 to 7. In this type of training it is fairly easy to maintain a moderate intensity of activity for an extended period of time with little chance of injury.

▶ **Aerobic Interval Training**
A series of alternate bouts of work and recovery where the intensity and duration of the work determines the intensity

and duration of the recovery period. Shorter periods of high intensity work lead to greater improvement in aerobic capacity.

▶ **Aerobic Circuit Training**
A form of aerobic work either extended (20 minutes) or repeated (10 minutes) followed by a number of different muscular exercises. This type of training has the two-fold benefit of improving aerobic fitness while increasing muscular strength and endurance.

Unique benefit. Work of higher intensity leads to greater improvement in aerobic capacity. For example, you are probably not able to run a 5 minute mile without stopping. If you wanted to train at that intensity, however, you could run on a treadmill at a 5 minute per mile pace for 15 seconds and then rest for 30 seconds. If you repeated that cycle of running 15 seconds and resting 30 seconds 20 times, you would have completed a 5 minute mile—but it would take you 14 minutes and 30 seconds to do it! With interval training, the benefits come during the work period as your body learns to "buffer" lactic acid and over time can even store greater amounts of the anaerobic enzymes necessary for higher intensity training. The recovery period is just as important, because it allows your body to rebuild the enzymes used during the work period and remove lactic acid from the muscles so you can continue training. Interval training is ideal for healthy persons interested in improving performance and being able to train at higher exercise intensities. The trade-off comes with the higher risk of injury associated with higher intensity training.

AEROBIC CIRCUIT TRAINING

In aerobic circuit training, some form of aerobic work is alternated with some form of resistance training. The purpose of aerobic circuit training is to improve both aerobic fitness and muscular strength and endurance. Circuit classes usually involve one extended (20+ minutes) or repeated bouts (10 minutes) of aerobic dance exercise followed by a number of different muscular exercises. The muscular exercises should be set up to provide overload, challenging the targeted muscle groups to work to fatigue. This can be accomplished by increasing the amount of resistance provided or by increasing the number of repetitions. Using light weights (1 to 3 pounds) for brief time periods most likely represents an "underload" and will not result in improved muscular strength or endurance.

There are numerous ways to set up aerobic circuits, with various advantages and disadvantages to each. Most forms of aerobic circuit training involve an aerobic dance segment (of varying length) combined with any number of exercise stations. To maximize the time it takes to move away from aerobics to the established stations, most instructors lead an extended aerobic segment (15+ minutes) followed by a number of different exercises. At the stations, you might perform an exercise for a certain number of repetitions or a specified period of time before moving on to the next station or exercise. Allowing only a predetermined amount of time for each station allows you to work at your own pace, ensures that you will complete each station on the circuit, and keeps the class organized. Specifying the number of repetitions to be finished before changing exercises or stations still allows you to self-pace your workout, but does not ensure that you will get through all the stations in the allotted time.

The exercises can be combined in a number of ways, such as focusing on opposing muscle groups or "super setting" by working one muscle group with three different exercises. Several examples of circuit workouts are presented in Figure 8-3.

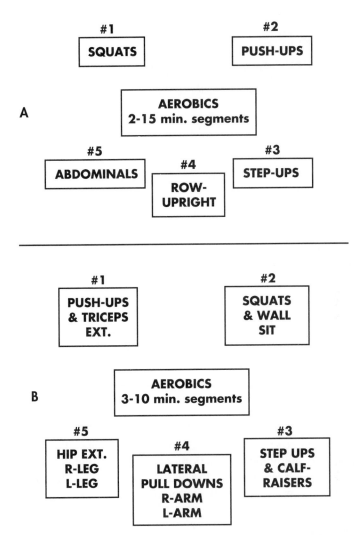

FIGURE 8-3   **A**, Warm-up; 15-minute aerobic segment followed by five 1-minute stations. Repeat 2 or 3 times for a 40- to 60-minute workout; cool down. **B**, Warm-up; 10-minute aerobic segment followed by five 1-minute stations, 2 exercises (30 seconds each) per station; repeat 3 times for a 45-minute workout; cool down.

POST AEROBIC COOL DOWN PHASE

Fitness Tip

Post Aerobic Cool Down Phase

G	Gradual
R	Reduced
A	Action
C	Control
E	Energized

Purpose. To gradually return the body close to normal or resting state after exertion. The accompanying Fitness Tip outlines the GRACE sequence for this phase.

Plan. Think of this exercise segment as the physiologic opposite of the warm-up. The keys are still in the ignition, the car is still running, but the engine is idling.

THINK *G*RADUAL

Just as you should not start suddenly, do not stop suddenly. Gradually reducing heart rate and breathing allows your body to begin reversing all the metabolic processes put in gear by your workout. It takes several minutes or longer for this to happen. During this period and throughout the remainder of the workout your body continues to slowly recover.

THINK *R*EDUCED

Use the slower-paced movements of the post aerobic cool down to let yourself begin to relax and enjoy the satisfaction of having completed the aerobic segment. Focus on breathing deeply, using the abdominal muscles (diaphragmatic breathing) and begin to prepare mentally for the upcoming muscle work.

THINK *A*CTION

Unlike the faster pace of the aerobic phase, the intensity in this segment will be very similar to the warm-up. You will begin to decrease the intensity and amount of movement with the lower body, but you will still be using both the upper and lower body continuously. Instructors often repeat movements from the aerobic segment here because you have already learned the patterns and can perform them easily and safely. This post aerobic cool down can also serve as a bridge to the muscular strength and endurance segment, using large-muscle, multi-joint movements, such as the squat, mixed with other low-intensity aerobic work.

THINK **C**ONTROL

Muscular control is essential at this point in the workout. Continue to perform movements through a full but controlled range of motion, modifying when necessary.

THINK **E**NERGIZED

Now is the time to give yourself a mental pat on the back and think about getting a drink of water if you haven't already. You should be sweaty as you begin to cool down (if you are not it means you need to either drink more water or work harder)—but you'll also be energized and ready to move on!

MUSCULAR WORK

Purpose.   To increase muscular strength or endurance or both.

Plan.   The majority of muscular work in the post aerobic segment provides an opportunity to improve both muscular strength and endurance. Overload is provided by working against increasing amounts of resistance or performing a greater number of repetitions. You can increase the overload in a number of ways. Consider an abdominal curl. The basic curl is biomechanically easiest when performed with the hands by the body (Figure 8-4) or the chest (Figure 8- 5); having the hands supporting or cradling the head is an intermediate level (Figures 8-6 and 8-7); and having them extended beyond the head is an advanced, more difficult position (Figure 8-8). You could also provide overload by using the lower body with a posterior tilt into a reverse curl (Figure 8-9); performing more crunches; or varying the abdominal muscles used (Figure 8-10) as well as the range of motion of a particular activity (Figure 8-11). Other options include increasing or decreasing the speed of movement or angle of contraction (Figure 8-12) or adding external resistance (such as a body ball) or providing self- resistance with the hands (Figure 8-13). Virtually any muscle group can be overloaded by applying these principles.

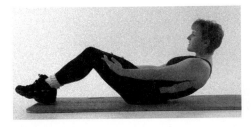

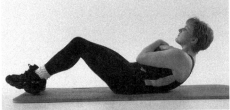

FIGURE 8-4   Basic curl with the hands by the body.

FIGURE 8-5   Basic curl with the hands over the chest.

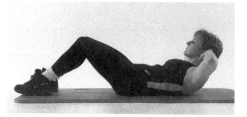

FIGURE 8-6 Intermediate level: curl with hands supporting the head.

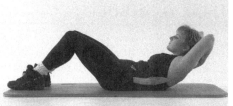

FIGURE 8-7 Intermediate level: curl with hands cradling the head.

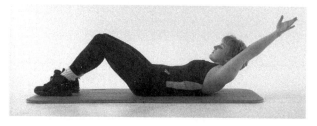

FIGURE 8-8 Advanced level: curl with hands beyond the head is an advanced position.

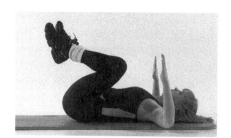

FIGURE 8-9 You can work to overload by using the lower body with a posterior tilt into a reverse curl.

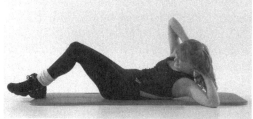

FIGURE 8-10 Performing more crunches or varying the abdominal muscles used will help you achieve overload.

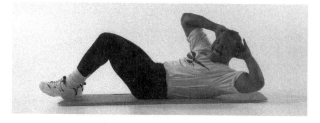

FIGURE 8-11 Increasing the range of motion of a particular activity is another way to achieve overload.

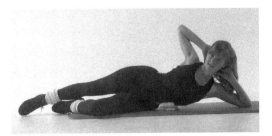

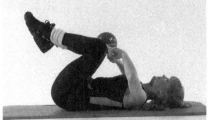

FIGURE 8-12 Other options on the progression toward overload are to increase or decrease the speed of movement or angle of contraction.

FIGURE 8-13 Adding external resistance or resistance with the hands will help achieve overload, too.

By targeting the major muscle groups, dance exercise classes can promote functional strength and endurance to enhance your ability to complete everyday tasks without fatigue. Muscle groups that are not used very much need to be strengthened, and those that are used extensively need to be stretched. (See Figure 8-14 on the following page.)

FINAL COOL DOWN AND STATIC STRETCHING

Purpose. To return the body to resting state and improve flexibility of the joints and muscular system. The Fitness Tip Below offers tips for the final cool down.

Plan. By this point in the workout, heart rate and breathing should have returned to near normal levels. The final cool down consists mainly of seated or standing stretching of the muscle groups used throughout the workout. Ideally, the stretching segment improves flexibility, potentially reducing the risk of later injury caused by shortened or tight muscles.

Fitness Tip

Guidelines for the Final Cool Down

Static Stretching: stretch and hold = SAFE

Ballistic Stretching: stretch with bouncing = NOT SAFE

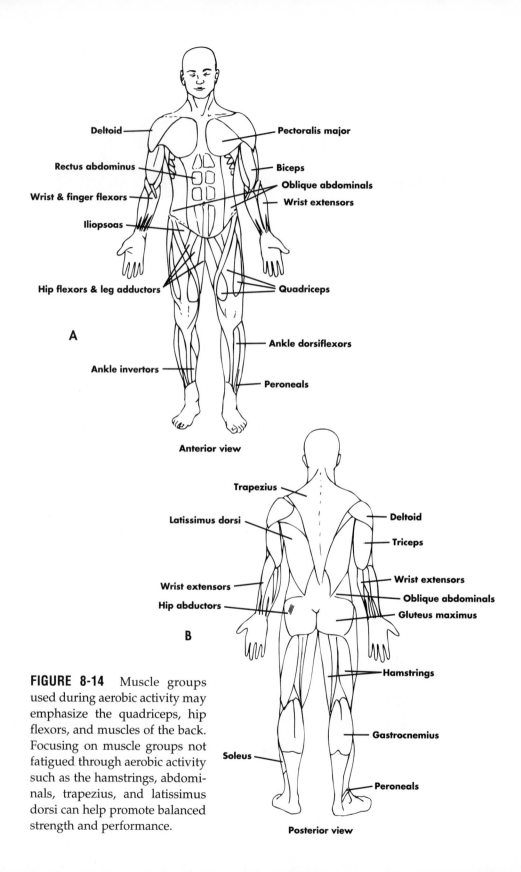

FIGURE 8-14 Muscle groups used during aerobic activity may emphasize the quadriceps, hip flexors, and muscles of the back. Focusing on muscle groups not fatigued through aerobic activity such as the hamstrings, abdominals, trapezius, and latissimus dorsi can help promote balanced strength and performance.

Two of the different stretching techniques often used during the final cool down include **ballistic** and **static stretching**. Many persons are accustomed to bouncing while they stretch, usually in the hope that they will be able to stre———tch the muscle further by forcing it. This ballistic stretching is overload in a dangerous sense! When you subject a muscle to sudden or excessive force, the muscle responds by reflexively contracting. This phenomenon, called the stretch reflex, is simply a built-in protective mechanism to keep the muscle from overstretching and injury. Static stretching, by comparison, overcomes the stretch reflex by applying a controlled, manageable force and holding the stretch at that point. Rather than repeatedly tugging on the muscle, a static stretch gently stretches the muscle and coaxes it to lengthen a bit. To produce a lasting change in the resting length of a muscle, you should try to hold any stretch for an extended period of time: ideally 20 to 45 seconds. More details and specific stretches for different muscle groups are presented in Chapter 11.

SUMMARY

- The warm-up, recommended before participation in any fitness activity, is key to getting your body prepared to exercise.
- The GRACE principle will help your body prepare for and recover from your aerobic workout.
- To improve aerobic fitness, ACSM guidelines recommend a training zone of 5 to 7 on the RPE scale and expending 300 Calories per workout.
- Aerobic steady state training, aerobic interval training and aerobic circuit training have unique benefits that you can use to create or vary a program to meet your personal fitness goals.
- Using the principle of overload, you can use your aerobic workout to increase muscular strength and endurance. You can vary your routine to increase either repetitions or the amount of resistance of a particular exercise.
- Static stretching is an important part of the cool down phase and helps your body return to a resting state.

▶ **Ballistic Stretching**
Quick, repetitive stretches using bouncing motions that could result in injury.

▶ **Static Stretching**
A controlled process of "stretch and hold" that safely and effectively increases range of motion with little chance of injury.

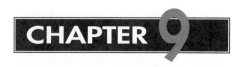

CHAPTER 9

YOUR ACTION PLAN:
DEVELOPING
AEROBIC FITNESS

OBJECTIVES

After reading this chapter, you should be able to do the following:

- Determine what makes your aerobic class "aerobic."
- Apply the ACSM guidelines for developing and maintaining fitness to your personal action plan.
- Distinguish between the different methods for estimating exercise intensity.
- Use the rating of perceived exertion (RPE) to predict your exercise intensity.
- Understand the need for physical activity in improving your health-related components of fitness.

KEY TERMS

While reading this chapter, you will become familiar with the following terms:

▶ Maximal Heart Rate (MHR) ▶ Talk Test
▶ Rating of Perceived Exertion (RPE)

WHAT MAKES YOUR AEROBICS CLASS "AEROBIC?"

In simple terms, *aerobic* refers to the dominant use of the aerobic energy systems during an activity or workout. Saying that you are working aerobically implies that you are supplying your body with enough oxygen to meet the demand for oxygen. *Anaerobic* means *without oxygen* and refers to the use of systems that don't require oxygen to produce energy.

> ## Aerobic and Anaerobic
>
> Most activities use a combination of aerobic and anaerobic energy.
>
> Aerobic = with oxygen
>
> Anaerobic = without oxygen

Being aerobic or anaerobic, however, is not like turning a light switch on or off. Most of your activities use energy provided by some combination of both the aerobic and anaerobic pathways (the box above summarizes the difference between the two). The aerobic energy system predominates when you are working at a level you can sustain for an extended period of time. Workouts like your aerobics class should improve your aerobic fitness and can improve body composition by helping you lose fat and maintain or even gain muscle. To review the ACSM guidelines for developing and maintaining aerobic fitness see the Fitness Tip below.

ACSM GUIDELINES

FREQUENCY (3 TO 5 DAYS PER WEEK)

Aerobic fitness improves with 3 or 4 days of training each week: after 3 days, your ability to improve aerobic fitness diminishes and the potential for injury increases. Aerobic fitness is not improved but may be maintained with 1 or 2 days of exercise each week. There is no hard and fast rule or a "magic" number of workouts. How often you work out aerobically depends on your level of fitness, age, personal preference, and the other types of exercise you regularly engage in.

Fitness Tip

> ## ACSM Guidelines for Developing and Maintaining Fitness
>
> To affect fitness related changes in your life, use the following guidelines:
>
> Frequency = 3 to 5 days a week
>
> Duration = 20 to 60 minutes
>
> Intensity = somewhat hard to hard

Recommendation. Start with 3 or 4 days a week and maintain that level for 4 to 6 weeks. This will give you a chance to get over the initial soreness of exercise and to develop a base level of aerobic fitness, muscular strength, and endurance. After this initial training period you may want to add additional workouts for enjoyment or increased caloric expenditure, or you may want to maintain your fitness at that level. Use a variety of activities with different impact levels to reduce your risk of sustaining an injury that would keep you from exercising. Listen to your body: when you come to work out you should feel that you have lots of energy—and leave the workout feeling even better.

INTENSITY AND DURATION (SOMEWHAT HARD TO HARD FOR 20 TO 60 MINUTES)

The intensity and the duration of exercise are so interrelated that you really cannot talk about one without considering the other. Intensity and duration have what is called an inverse relationship: as one goes up the other usually goes down and vice versa. To improve aerobic fitness, the higher the intensity the shorter the duration of exercise; the lower the intensity, the longer the workout should be. For example, 15 minutes of very high intensity work (90% to 95% maximum aerobic capacity) has been shown to increase aerobic fitness, although most persons could not maintain such a high intensity for any length of time. At the other extreme, very low intensity work performed for long periods of time may be best for certain special populations because of the low risk of injury or other complications. For most healthy persons, though, the workout design should be tailored to meet individual needs and goals. If aerobic fitness is the primary goal, try to challenge the aerobic system by working longer and or harder or both. If you are interested in weight control you will want to make sure that you are expending 200 to 300 calories per session—and you can vary the duration of the workout accordingly. When comparing workouts for weight loss, you will see about the same results from a variety of different workouts *if* you expend the same number of calories.

Recommendation. Moderate- to high-intensity exercise performed for about 30 to 45 minutes.

MONITORING EXERCISE INTENSITY

The best way to know how hard you are working is to measure how much oxygen your muscles are consuming, but this technique requires a laboratory and expensive equipment. Other means of predicting (rather than actually measuring) exercise intensity include the use of **rating of perceived exertion (RPE), heart rate,** and the **talk test.**

RATING OF PERCEIVED EXERTION

RPE is a tool to measure your perception of exercise intensity during a workout. Research has shown that RPE correlates well with oxygen consumption and is accurate for most exercisers, whether they are at an advanced or beginning level. As you exercise, you match how you feel to a chart that has verbal descriptors of exercise intensity linked with corresponding numbers.

There are two scales in widespread use. The first scale rates exercise from 1 to 19 and is based on some of the earliest research in this area (Table 9-1). The one we will use in class is a bit more user friendly, with a scale ranging from 1 to 10 (Table 9-2).

TABLE 9-1
Original Rating of Perceived Exertion

How Does the Exercise Feel?	Category RPE Scale
	6
Very, very light	7
	8
Very light	9
	10
Fairly light	11
	12
Somewhat hard	13
	14
Hard	15
	16
Very hard	17
	18
Very, very hard	19
	20

From Borg GA: Psychophysical basis of perceived exertion, Med Sci Sports Exerc 14:377, 1982. Copyright American College of Sports Medicine, Williams & Wilkins Publishing Company.

TABLE 9-2
Optional Rating of Perceived Exertion

How Does the Exercise Feel?	Category–Ratio RPE Scale,
Nothing at all	0
Very, very weak	0.5
Very weak	1
Weak	2
Moderate	3
Somewhat strong	4
Strong	5
	6
Very strong	7
	8
	9
Very, very strong	10
Maximal	

From Borg GA: Psychophysical basis of perceived exertion, Med Sci Sports Exerc 14:377, 1982. Copyright American College of Sports Medicine, Williams & Wilkins Publishing Company.

▶ **Rating of Perceived Exertion (RPE)**
A scale that takes into account how you feel to measure the intensity of a workout. Although this is a subjective scale, research shows that this method is accurate for most exercisers whether at the advanced or beginner level.

▶ **Maximal Heart Rate (MHR)**
The highest heart rate a person can attain, which is affected by age and genetics.

▶ **Talk Test**
A nonscientific method that uses your breathing and ability to talk to gauge exercise intensity.

As found on Table 9-2, if you feel that you are working at a very *light pace*, you would be about 2 or 3 (*weak to moderate*) on the RPE scale and feel that you could keep going for an extended period of time. If you are overexerting and unable to continue, you'd be at 10 (*very, very strong*) and working very, very hard!

Much of your workout should take place at the *somewhat hard* level (4 to 6: *somewhat strong* to *strong*). At this level you will be warm and perspiring, but not gasping for breath. If you push into the hard range (7 to 9: *very strong*), your fitness level will probably determine how long you can continue. In the *hard* range, breathing becomes more difficult; if fatigue builds you may need to slow down to maintain proper form and technique. By adjusting the intensity up or down on the basis of how you feel, you can personalize your aerobic workout to make sure you are working at an appropriate pace to see improvement.

Assessment 9-1 at the end of this chapter is a summary form you can use to track the intensity and duration of your workouts over a 6-week period. Complete the form to evaluate the intensity of your workout once a week. Completing the form on the same day each week at the same time will be useful in tracking your progress.

HEART RATE

The use of heart rate to predict exercise intensity is also widely used in aerobic dance exercise. However, the "prescribed" exercise heart rate is based on your predicted **maximal heart rate (MHR)**. Because MHR is predicted with a formula based on averages rather than being measured individually, it will be accurate for some but not for others: your predicted heart rate may be too high or low for you. Other considerations, such as making sure you have counted correctly for the proper amount of time and the fact that you have to stop exercising to take your heart rate make it a less than precise means of monitoring exercise intensity. A number of research studies have also demonstrated that heart rates over-predict exercise intensity in aerobic dance exercise routines. Because of these problems with exercise heart rate, we recommend using RPE instead.

TALK TEST

The so-called "talk test" uses your breathing rate to gauge exercise intensity. Talking should be easy during the warm-up; become more difficult because of faster breathing as the workout continues; and become easy again during the cool down and stretching. Although you do not have to actually talk to determine whether you can, it sometimes helps to ask yourself if you could, especially during the aerobic segment. If you could chatter away as though you are taking a stroll in the park, you probably need to pick up the pace a bit. If you would be unable to talk or could only gasp out a "yes" or a "no" to your neighbor, you are probably working too hard and should ease off to a more manageable pace.

PHYSICAL ACTIVITY IN INCREASING HEALTH AND FITNESS

Exercise of lower intensity than mentioned above has been shown to improve general health and well-being and reduce the risk of developing certain disease conditions. If you are completely inactive, **health-related changes** can occur by simply becoming more active. Look for ways to incorporate exercise into the routine of every day, such as walking rather than riding the bus or parking your car farther away from a store rather than waiting for a close parking spot. If you are interested in improving your aerobic fitness level, though, your best bet is to follow the guidelines previously outlined.

INTERACTION OF FREQUENCY, INTENSITY, AND DURATION OF EXERCISE

It is difficult to discuss the relative benefits of varying exercise intensity, duration, and frequency to produce overload because of their interrelationship. Is one more important than the other in improving fitness? Without considering genetics, it appears that the intensity of exercise, rather than the duration or frequency of exercise, determines the amount of improvement in aerobic fitness (see the Fitness Tip below).

Exercise of moderate intensity and duration is generally a sufficient overload and results in improvement in fitness for most persons. High-intensity exercise, on the other hand, although appropriate for some, is linked with a higher injury and drop-out rate than low- to moderate-intensity training. Use your body as a guide when deciding how you should mix and match these variables: when you increase the intensity of your workout you usually cannot go quite as long, so you decrease the duration; if you plan on working aerobically for 60 minutes, decrease the intensity to a pace you can maintain for that period of time.

Fitness Tip

Duration and Intensity

If duration of exercise is fixed (as in aerobics class), *intensity* becomes the key variable to determine caloric expenditure.

Be sure to participate in aerobic classes that are at an appropriate level of intensity for your fitness level that will best help you achieve your personal fitness goals.

To determine the benefits of aerobic fitness, weight control, and preventive health maintenance, the most important factor appears to be the total amount of exercise performed. Something (ANYTHING!) is better than nothing. ACSM guidelines are intended for those interested in developing and/or maintaining aerobic fitness. Increasing frequency, intensity, or duration beyond these guidelines is not recommended for the general population.

SUMMARY

- Most physical activities combine aerobic and anaerobic pathways. Exercising for an extended period of time should improve your aerobic fitness, body composition, and help you to gain muscle.
- If you are just starting an exercise program you should train 3 or 4 days a week for 4 to 6 weeks before adding any additional workouts to your schedule.
- If you are interested in weight control, you should plan your exercise sessions to expend 200 to 300 Calories, and you can vary the duration of the workout accordingly.
- The rating of perceived exertion scale is an easy-to-use tool that measures the intensity of your workout and takes into account individual differences. It can be used to plan your workout sessions effectively and help you attain your fitness goals.
- Any form of physical activity is better than no physical activity.
- Increasing frequency, intensity, or duration beyond the ACSM guidelines is not recommended.

ASSESSMENT 9-1

Rating of Perceived Exertion Session Evaluation

Name _____ Section _____ Date _____

INSTRUCTIONS

Complete a section of this form to evaluate the intensity of your workout once a week. Completing the form on the same day each week at the same time will be useful in tracking your progress.

RATING OF PERCEIVED EXERTION

How Does the Exercise Feel?	Category RPE Scale
	6
Very, very light	7
	8
Very light	9
	10
Fairly light	11
	12
Somewhat hard	13
	14
Hard	15
	16
Very hard	17
	18
Very, very hard	19
	20

How Does the Exercise Feel?	Category–Ratio RPE Scale,
Nothing at all	0
Very, very weak	0.5
Very weak	1
Weak	2
Moderate	3
Somewhat strong	4
Strong	5
	6
Very strong	7
	8
	9
Very, very strong	10
Maximal	

Week 1

Date: _____

Time: _____

	Intensity Level	Duration (minutes)
Warm–up		
Aerobic Phase		
Post Aerobic Cool Down		
Muscular Work		
Final Cool Down/ Static Stretching		

Week 2

Date: _____

Time: _____

	Intensity Level	Duration (minutes)
Warm–up		
Aerobic Phase		
Post Aerobic Cool Down		
Muscular Work		
Final Cool Down/ Static Stretching		

Week 3	Intensity Level	Duration (minutes)
Date:		
Time:		
Warm–up		
Aerobic Phase		
Post Aerobic Cool Down		
Muscular Work		
Final Cool Down/ Static Stretching		

Week 4	Intensity Level	Duration (minutes)
Date:		
Time:		
Warm–up		
Aerobic Phase		
Post Aerobic Cool Down		
Muscular Work		
Final Cool Down/ Static Stretching		

Week 5	Intensity Level	Duration (minutes)
Date:		
Time:		
Warm–up		
Aerobic Phase		
Post Aerobic Cool Down		
Muscular Work		
Final Cool Down/ Static Stretching		

Week 6	Intensity Level	Duration (minutes)
Date:		
Time:		
Warm–up		
Aerobic Phase		
Post Aerobic Cool Down		
Muscular Work		
Final Cool Down/ Static Stretching		

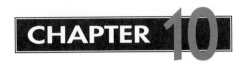

CHAPTER 10

YOUR ACTION PLAN: AEROBIC TECHNIQUE AND PROGRESSIONS

OBJECTIVES

After reading this chapter, you should be able to do the following:

- Maximize your oxygen consumption by focusing on the lower body muscles.
- Learn to use the upper part of your body to give you an added muscular strength and endurance workout.
- Modify select exercises to increase or decrease intensity to suit your particular needs.

KEY TERM

While reading this chapter, you will become familiar with the following term:

▶ **Personalize**

PUTTING YOUR PLAN INTO ACTION

Effective aerobic training can occur with various types of workouts. We described steady state, interval, and circuit training in Chapter 8 (they are summarized in the box below). Within each of these workout options you may need to find ways to increase or decrease exercise intensity. Each time you work out, remember to listen to your body and adjust the workout accordingly. It is helpful to know how to modify typical aerobic dance movements so that you can **personalize** any workout to meet your needs. We have selected some movements used in most aerobic dance exercise classes to analyze and offer intensity modifications. Most of those chosen are similar to other movements and the modifications will be similar. You should make every effort to remain posturally correct throughout the workout by maintaining correct posture and using the abdominal muscles to stabilize your trunk or torso.

FOCUS: THE LOWER BODY

The key to remember during aerobic dance exercise is to keep the lower body moving! It is the lower body that will consume large quantities of oxygen and make the workout aerobic; staying in one place and relying on vigorous arm pumping to elevate the heart rate will simply elevate the heart rate without significantly increasing oxygen consumption. The amount of oxygen you consume determines the number of calories you expend, so to increase caloric expenditure you will want to focus on the larger, lower body muscles that consume more oxygen. Higher intensity exercise burns more calories than lower intensity exercise, but that does not mean that the high intensity modifications are for everyone. As you increase exercise intensity, you potentially increase risk of injury because of higher impact forces and possible fatigue. Work at the exercise intensity that is right for *you*—and modify movements when you need to.

Using the upper body can improve muscular endurance and keep the movements interesting and fun. If you feel that you are working too hard, drop your arms out of the movement for a while and concentrate on fully engaging the lower body (see Figure 10-2). The easiest use of the upper body occurs below the shoulders; as you increase the height of the movement the perception of intensity also increases. It is also common to have a burning sensation in the front or top of the

Types of Aerobic Training

Steady state = continuous work
Interval training = alternate work and recovery
Circuit training = combined aerobic and strength work

shoulders if you are performing movements using those same muscle groups repeatedly. Simply lowering the arms and performing similar movements while you keep the arms lower than the shoulders should reduce local muscle fatigue and allow you to continue. It may also be helpful to minimize upper body work when you are learning a new or complicated movement; add the arms back in the routine when you feel comfortable again.

Designing a workout that is right for you is key to your success. Use the Fitness Tip below to adapt your workout effectively.

VARYING EXERCISE INTENSITY

A number of exercises can be varied in intensity, either lower or higher. We have selected the following exercises for this section because together they make up a number of the most common movements found in today's aerobics classes: march in place (Figure 10-1), knee lift (Figure 10-2), step touch (Figure 10-3), jumping jack (Figure 10-4), step kick (Figure 10-5), rear lift on step (Figure 10-6), and side lift on step (Figure 10-7).

▶ **Personalize**
To make personal or individual; in this context it applies to the ways in which you can increase or decrease exercise intensity so that you can maximize results from the time you spend working out!

Text continued on p. 150

Fitness Tip

Effective Aerobic Training and Intensity Modification

Focus on the lower body!
Emphasize postural awareness and muscular control!

To Increase Intensity
-Increase the range of movement

-Increase the use of the lower and/or upper body

-Add propulsion

-Increase the speed of movement

To Reduce Intensity
-Make the movement smaller

-Decrease use of the upper and/or lower body

-Remove impact

-Decrease the speed of movement

A   B   C

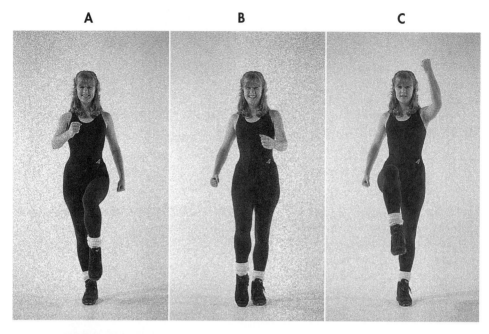

FIGURE 10-1 **A,** March in place. **B,** Low intensity. **C,** High Intensity.

A   B   C

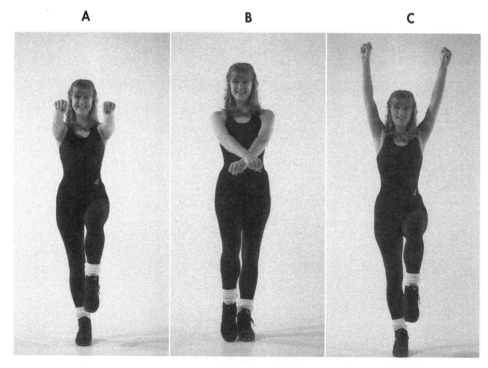

FIGURE 10-2 **A,** Knee lift. **B,** Low intensity. **C,** High Intensity.

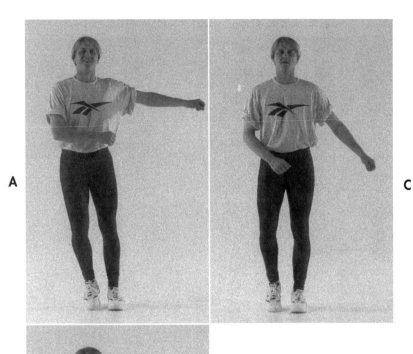

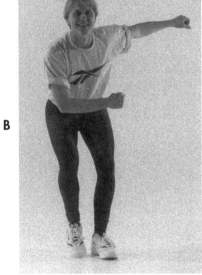

FIGURE 10-3 **A**, Step touch. **B**, Low intensity. **C**, High Intensity.

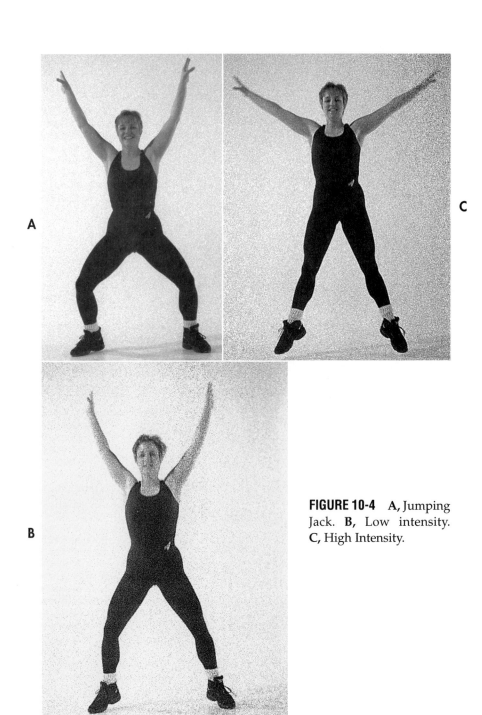

FIGURE 10-4 **A,** Jumping Jack. **B,** Low intensity. **C,** High Intensity.

A

B

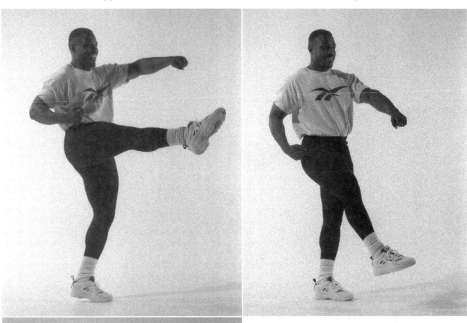

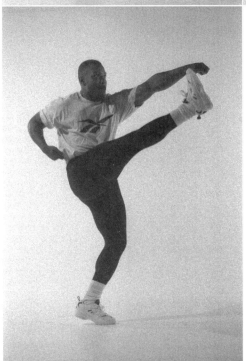

FIGURE 10-5 **A,** Step kick. **B,** Low intensity. **C,** High Intensity.

C

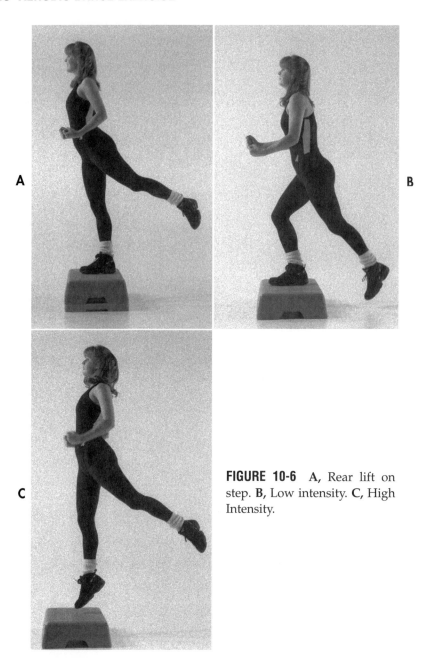

FIGURE 10-6 **A**, Rear lift on step. **B**, Low intensity. **C**, High Intensity.

A   B

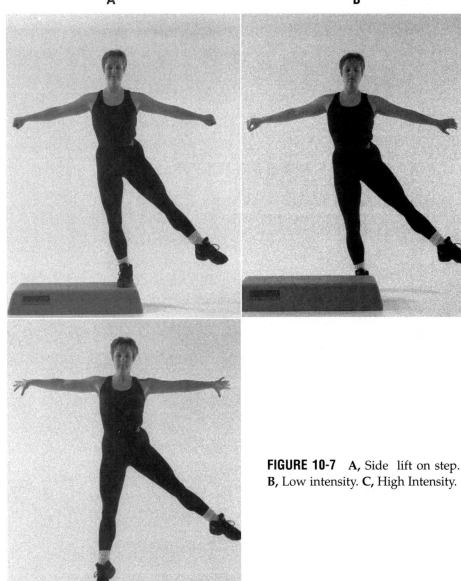

FIGURE 10-7 **A,** Side lift on step.
B, Low intensity. **C,** High Intensity.

C

SUMMARY

- The key to maximizing oxygen consumption and energy expenditure is to keep the lower body moving.
- Staying in one place and relying on vigorous arm pumping to elevate heart rate simply elevates heart rate without significantly increasing oxygen consumption.
- Adding upper body movements to an existing routine will give you added muscular strength and endurance benefits.
- A slight burning sensation is normal in the front or top of your shoulders if you are performing movements using those same muscle groups repeatedly.

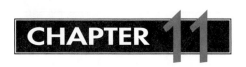
YOUR ACTION PLAN: FLEXIBILITY TECHNIQUES AND PROGRESSIONS

OBJECTIVES

After reading this chapter, you should be able to do the following:

- Relate the role of balanced flexibility to proper body alignment.
- Understand the relationship between flexibility and strength and explain how the two work together to help you perform your daily activities.
- Apply the five principles of flexibility training to create permanent changes in your connective tissues.
- Focus on the correct way to stretch at low intensity for long duration.
- Effectively perform a range of flexibility exercises for each muscle group, complete with variations for increasing or decreasing intensity.

KEY TERMS

While reading this chapter, you will become familiar with the following terms:

- ▶ Connective Tissue
- ▶ Elastic Quality of Connective Tissues
- ▶ Flexibility
- ▶ Plastic Quality of Connective Tissues

BALANCED FLEXIBILITY

Balanced flexibility is just as important to your appearance and health as muscular strength or aerobic fitness. **Inflexibility** is often the cause of chronic pain in daily life and acute injury in sports and other activities. It can also limit strength potential because it prevents movement through the complete range of motion. Flexibility must be an integral part of a balanced fitness program.

Balanced flexibility is crucial to proper body alignment. Good alignment and posture affect not only how you look and how you feel emotionally but also how you are perceived by other people. Think of the posture of a depressed, insecure, or disinterested person. Then picture the alignment of a confident, competent person. Balanced strength and flexibility for posture affects much more than your physical fitness scores.

Tight muscles pull the spine and other joints out of neutral alignment. Tight hip muscles can pull the lower back out of alignment and thereby cause chronic lower back pain. They can also cause problems "up the line" as the chest, shoulders, and head also move out of alignment to compensate for the back position.

Another common area of decreased flexibility is in the chest and shoulders; restricted motion here can cause the shoulders to round forward. Rounded shoulders may then cause your head to jut forward. This poor alignment can cause uneven wear-and-tear on the joints, back and neck pain, and even seemingly unrelated conditions such as carpal tunnel syndrome.

INDIVIDUAL DIFFERENCES

Flexibility is variable from person to person and from joint to joint in the same person. The amount of flexibility needed also varies from person to person, depending on the person's activities. For example, a dancer may need extreme hamstring flexibility to perform a high kick without injury. A gymnast may require extreme shoulder and back flexibility to perform routines on the parallel bars. Those extremes of motion are not needed and may not be desirable for those outside specialized sports.

COMBINE STRENGTH TRAINING WITH STRETCHING

Those with extreme flexibility also need the strength to support it. Sometimes ex-gymnasts and dancers experience pain and joint instability if they do not maintain muscular strength later in life.

Aim for both strength and flexibility that will allow you to maintain a neutral posture and perform the activities of your daily life without undue strain or fatigue.

STRETCH FOR STRESS REDUCTION

Stretching itself can also have a positive effect on your state of mind and emotions. By focusing on the relaxation and stretching of tense muscles, you will find that your mind can also relax and focus. Stretching is an important element of stress reduction.

HOW TO STRETCH EFFECTIVELY

When training for flexibility, you are stretching primarily **connective tissue**. This connective tissue is located around and between the muscle fibers, eventually converging to form the tendons that connect the muscle fibers to the bones.

Connective tissue possesses qualities that act like elastic and qualities that act like plastic. As you know, when elastic is stretched, it returns to its original resting length when the stretch is released. Think of an elastic waistband: it can stretch then immediately return to the shortened position. However, when plastic is stretched it stays in the stretched position even after the stretching force is removed. A change in length of a piece of elastic is temporary; a change in length of a piece of plastic is permanent.

When you stretch lightly before an activity, you address the **elastic quality of muscle and connective tissue**; no lasting change occurs. Such short duration stretches take the muscles through their full length and range of motion to help decrease stiffness and prepare them for the upcoming activity. Such brief, pre-activity stretches will not permanently increase your flexibility.

THE FIVE PRINCIPLES OF PERMANENT CHANGE

True flexibility training seeks to make changes in the **plastic qualities of connective tissue.** Plastic changes are permanent changes in length that will remain

▶ **Inflexibility**
Decreased ability to move through a joint's full range of motion. It can cause chronic pain in daily life and increase chance of injury in sports or physical activity while limiting strength potential by preventing movement through a full range of motion.

▶ **Connective Tissue**
Located around and between muscle fibers, these tissues connect muscle fibers to the bones.

▶ **Elastic Quality of Connective Tissues**
The ability of connective tissues to stretch and then return to a previously shortened position like an elastic band, enhanced by light stretching.

▶ **Plastic Quality of Connective Tissue**
The ability of connective tissue to change permanently in length.

after the training session. To make safe and lasting changes in the length of connective tissue, certain principles must be applied.

First. The tissues must be warm. A temperature of 103° to 104° is most conducive to permanent changes, so do not expect to improve your flexibility if you stretch without a thorough warm-up.

Second. The most effective stretches are of a low intensity and long duration. The muscle tissue must relax before the force is applied to the connective tissue. So, to stretch effectively, come to the point of resistance—a sensation of stretch, not pain. Hold the stretch as you breathe deeply from three to five times. The deep breaths can enhance muscle relaxation. They also serve as a convenient method of

Guidelines for Flexibility Technique and Progression

1. Wear appropriate exercise apparel, either leotard and tights or loose-fitting shorts and T-shirt.
2. Warm-up adequately before performing the more intense stretches required for flexibility training. Muscles, tendons, and ligaments respond best when they are warm. Warm-up can be achieved by a rhythmic sequence of active movement for 3 to 5 minutes. You should feel as warm during stretching as you do when you begin cardiovascular training.
3. Hold a stretch for three to five deep, full breaths. Three to five breaths take 30 to 45 seconds. Deep breathing also helps to relax and release muscular tension.
4. Hold a stretch at the point of resistance, not the point of pain. Aim to relax the muscle by consistent tension and deep breathing so that further stretch can occur. Pain will increase muscle tension and defeat your efforts.
5. Stretch joints of the arms and legs with the spine in neutral alignment. Neutral alignment during the stretch will not only show you more clearly where you need to stretch, but also enable you to stretch safely without risk to other body parts.
6. If possible, stretch the right side, then the left side, then both sides simultaneously.
7. When possible, isometrically contract the muscle opposite the one being stretched. For example, contract the quadriceps (front thigh) muscle when stretching the hamstrings (back of the thigh). Contraction of the opposite muscle group may enhance relaxation of the muscle to be stretched.
8. Be content to work within your personal flexibility limits. Do not compare yourself with others in the class. Avoid trying to fake positions of extreme flexibility.

timing the duration of the stretch. The recommended duration for a stretch varies among experts, but a duration of 30 to 60 seconds is commonly recommended.

Third.   Contracting the muscle opposite the group to be stretched can help to relax the stretching muscle. As the opposite group contracts, your brain sends a message to the stretching muscle to relax.

Fourth.   Stretch individual areas with the full body in mind. Keep the spine in neutral position and the other body parts in safely aligned positions to avoid injury and to stretch evenly.

Fifth.   Stretching is most effective when it is performed every day. Part of the flexibility action plan might be to stretch daily, even when you are not in class.

Keep the guidelines in the accompanying box in mind when working to increase your flexibility in and outside your dance-exercise class.

MUSCLE GROUPS TO STRETCH

As with strength training, balance is a priority in stretching. Seek balanced flexibility on the right and left sides of the body, and in each motion around each joint.

Some areas of the body tend to be tighter than others, particularly if you sit most of the day. On the other hand, some muscles, such as those of the middle back and the shoulder blades may be overstretched in the person who sits all day or who stands in poor alignment. Do not spend time stretching muscles that are over-stretched already.

In choosing where to spend your flexibility time, refer to the results of your flexibility assessments in Chapter 3. Then spend the time available on the areas of tightness.

The following section of techniques and progressions will show a stretch for each muscle group and variations to increase or decrease the intensity of the stretch as necessary.

You may find that your flexibility varies from day to day. If you are experiencing mental stress, if you are dehydrated, if you ran several miles or performed some other vigorous activity the day before, you may feel tighter than on a previous day. Work at the appropriate intensity, which may vary slightly from day to day.

TECHNIQUES AND PROGRESSIONS

► LOWER BACK: KNEES TO CHEST

Lie face up on the floor. Lift the knees toward the chest one at a time and grasp the backs of the thighs with your hands. Separate the knees slightly and pull both knees upward toward your arm pits. The hips should lift slightly from the floor (Figure 11-1, *A*). The stretch is felt in the lower back. Hold the stretch for three to five breaths.

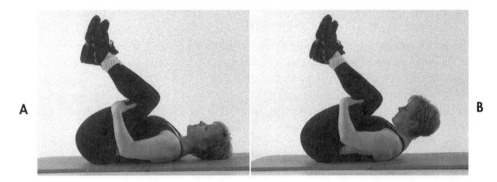

A   B

FIGURE 11-1 **A,** Lower back: knees to chest. **B,** To increase intensity lift your head, tucking your chin toward your chest.

Increase intensity: Perform the base action, then lift your head, tucking your chin toward your chest (Figure 11-1, *B*). This will stretch all the muscles along either side of your spine.

Decrease intensity: Stretch one leg at a time. Pull upward toward the chest until you feel a gentle stretch in the muscles next to your spine on that side.

▶ UPPER TORSO: SUPPORTED TORSO EXTENSION

Lie face down on the floor with forearms flat and elbows positioned beneath the shoulder joints. Keep both front hip bones in contact with the floor. Press the elbows and forearms against the floor and press the shoulder blades down and together to lengthen the distance between the ears and the shoulders. Lift the sternum upward to feel a stretch in the upper portion of the abdominals (Figure 11-2, *A*). Hold the stretch for three to five breaths.

Increase intensity: Press upward by partially straightening the elbows. Keep the shoulders pressed down and sternum lifted to stretch the upper abdominal area. Roll the shoulders outward and pull the shoulder blades together. Contract the buttocks and point the toes. There should not be discomfort in the lower back. If it is uncomfortable for you, make sure the sternum is lifted and shoulders are square. If discomfort persists, choose a position of reduced intensity by lowering the upper body.

Decrease intensity: Lift the upper torso so that the sternum clears the floor (Figure 11-2, *B*).

▶ HIP FLEXORS: LUNGE WITH PELVIC TILT

Stand in a slight forward lunge position with the back heel lifted and the knee relaxed. Contract the abdominals to tilt the pelvis backward to feel a stretch along the front of the hip of the rear leg. (In a backward pelvic tilt, the top of the pelvis moves backward and the pubic bone moves forward. It is like tilting a bucket to pour liquid out the back.) Hold the stretch for three to five deep breaths, increasing the stretch as you feel the muscles relax (Figure 11-3, *A*). Repeat with the opposite leg.

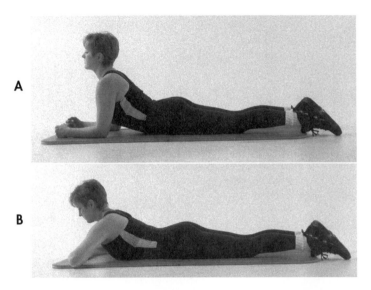

FIGURE 11-2 A, Upper torso: supported torso extension. **B,** To decrease intensity only lift the sternum so that it clears the floor.

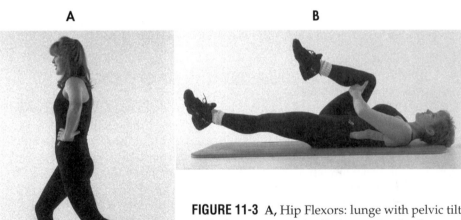

FIGURE 11-3 A, Hip Flexors: lunge with pelvic tilt. **B,** To decrease intensity lie face up on the floor and hug one knee toward your chest. Extend the opposite leg

Increase intensity: Start with a deeper bend of the forward knee and lift the arm on the same side as the hip to be stretched. Reach overhead and to the opposite side to feel the stretch higher along the hip flexor muscles.

Decrease intensity: Lie face up on the floor. Hug one knee toward your chest. Extend the opposite leg and let gravity gently stretch the front of the hip (Figure 11-3, *B*).

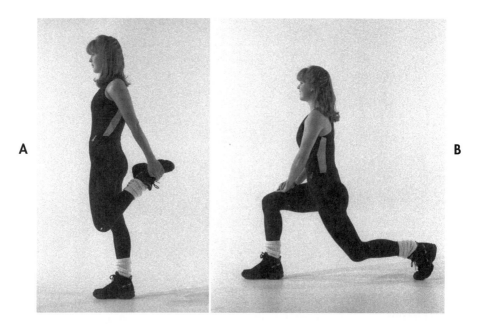

A

B

FIGURE 11-4 A, Quadriceps stretch: tilt pelvis backward with the abdominals and press the left thigh back to feel a stretch along the front of the left thigh. **B,** To increase intensity assume the lunge position with the pelvis tilted back and the right foot forward. Lower the left knee toward the floor until a stretch is felt along the front of the thigh.

▶ QUADRICEPS (FRONT THIGH): TILT WITH HIP EXTENSION

Touch the wall if you need to for balance. Stand on the right leg and grasp the left ankle with the left hand. Tilt your pelvis backward (like pouring water out of the bucket behind you) by strongly contracting and holding with your abdominal muscles. Keep the pelvis tilted by holding with the abdominals and press the left thigh back to feel a stretch along the front of the left thigh (Figure 11-4, *A*). Hold the stretch for three to five breaths.

Increase intensity: Assume a lunge position with the pelvis tilted back and the right foot forward. Lower the left (back) knee toward the floor (Figure 11-4, *B*) until a stretch is felt along the front of the thigh (quadriceps muscle).

Decrease intensity: Touch the wall for assistance with balance if needed. Stand upright with a neutral spine. Flex the right knee and grasp the right foot behind you. Press the right knee back so that the right thigh is parallel with the left knee. Do not allow the back to arch.

▶ HAMSTRINGS (REAR THIGH): STANDING HAMSTRING STRETCH WITH TILT

Place your right foot forward on a step or platform with the foot relaxed and the knee straight. Flex forward *from the hip*, keeping a slight inward curve at the lower back. The spine should not arch upward (Figure 11-5, *A*). Support your torso with

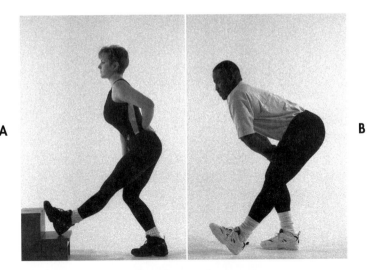

FIGURE 11-5 A, Hamstrings (rear thigh): standing hamstring stretch. **B,** To decrease intensity use the same standing position with the foot of the extended leg on the floor, not elevated on a step.

your arms on the standing leg. Move the top back of the legs toward the ceiling to feel a stretch along the rear thigh (hamstrings) of the right foot. Change legs and repeat the sequence to stretch the left hamstrings.

Increase intensity: Same position as described above, plus curl your tailbone toward the ceiling and your navel toward the front of the thigh. Gently rotate the extended leg inward and outward to stretch the inner and outer hamstrings.

Decrease intensity: Again, same initial standing position with the foot on the floor, not elevated on a step (Figure 11-5, *B*).

▶ HIP ABDUCTORS (OUTER HIP): MIDLINE HIP TWIST

To stretch the right side, lie face up on the floor with the left foot on the floor, knee flexed. Cross the right knee over the left. Hold the right ankle with the left hand and rotate the hip to feel a stretch along the outer rear of the right hip (Figure 11-6, *A*). Hold for three to five breaths. Repeat on the opposite side, crossing the left thigh over the right.

Increase intensity: Lift the left knee, hold the left ankle, and press the right thigh closer to your chest (Figure 11-6, *B*).

Decrease intensity: Cross the right thigh over the left and lift toward your chest without rotating the hip with your hands.

▶ HIP ADDUCTORS (INNER THIGH): BUTTERFLY PRESS

Sit upright with the spine in neutral (slight inward curve at the lower back). Place soles of the feet together at the position where you can maintain the curve in your lower back (Figure 11-7, *A*). Do not try to force the feet closer: keep them

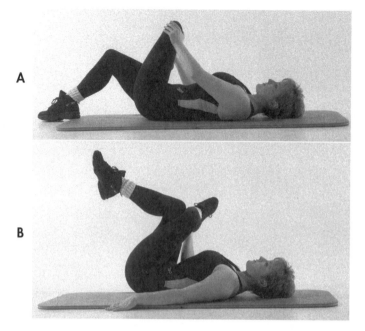

FIGURE 11-6 **A,** Hip abductors (outer hip): midline hip twist. **B,** To increase intensity lift the left knee, hold the left ankle, and press the right thigh closer to your chest. Note that the left knee is on top of the right knee.

where the back can stay straight. Do not allow the lower back to round backward as you stretch the inner thighs. Hold the stretch for three to five breaths. Keep your chest lifted.

Increase intensity: Same initial position, keeping your chest lifted and pulling the heels closer. Flex forward from the hip joints, leaning the torso toward the floor. Lift the sternum and press it forward past the feet, maintaining the inward curve at the lower back. Pull the knees down actively with the hip muscles.

Decrease intensity: Lean back slightly and support your upper body on your hands behind you (Figure 11-7, *B*). Press the knees down, one at a time, right then left.

▶ CALF WITH KNEE STRAIGHT (GASTROCNEMIUS): WALL STRETCH

Flex your right ankle as much as possible and place the ball of your right foot against a step or the wall, heel resting on the ground. Lean forward and press the right shin toward the step or wall with the knee straight to feel a stretch along the back of the calf. Actively contract the muscle along the front of your shin and hold the stretch for three to five breaths (Figure 11- 8, *A*). Repeat with the left calf.

Increase intensity: Stand on the edge of a step and slowly drop the right heel below the level of the step. Keep the right knee straight or soft; do not allow it to

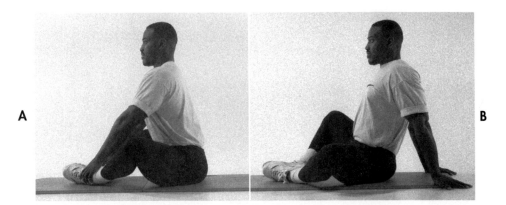

FIGURE 11-7 A, Hip adductors (inner thigh): butterfly with tilt. **B,** To increase intensity lean back slightly and support your upper body on your hands behind you. Press your knees down, one at a time, right, then left.

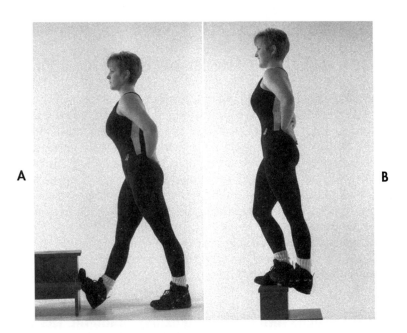

FIGURE 11-8 A, Calf with knee straight (gastrocnemius): wall stretch. **B,** To increase intensity stand on the edge of a step and slowly drop the right heel below the level of the step. Keep the right knee straight or soft; do not allow it to lock into hypertension.

lock into hyperextension (Figure 11-8, *B*). Hold the stretch for three to five breaths. Repeat with the left side.

Decrease intensity: Stand on the floor with your weight on the right leg (in a slight forward lunge position), knee slightly bent. Hold your left foot forward with toes pulled up. Lean forward from the hips to stretch your hamstrings and calf.

A   B

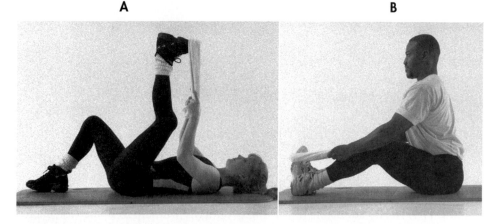

FIGURE 11-9 **A,** Calf with knee flexed (soleus): supine stretch with towel. **B,** To increase intensity assume a sitting position with the spine in neutral, knees flexed. Keep the sternum lifted and a slight inward curve to the lower back. Wrap a towel around the outsides of the feet and pull the forefeet toward the face.

▶ CALF WITH KNEE FLEXED (SOLEUS): SUPINE STRETCH WITH TOWEL

Lie face up on the floor with your right leg raised toward the ceiling and a towel around the forefoot. Maintain the right knee in a slightly flexed position. Pull the forefoot toward the floor to feel a stretch deep in the back of your calf. Hold for three to five breaths, contracting the muscle along the front of your shin (Figure 11-9, *A*).

Increase intensity: Same stretch sitting with the spine in neutral, knees flexed. Be sure to keep the sternum lifted and a slight inward curve at the lower back. Wrap a towel around the outside of the feet and pull the forefeet toward the face. Hold for three to five breaths, contracting the muscle along the front of your shin to actively pull the toes toward the face (Figure 11-9, *B*).

Decrease intensity: Stand in a slight forward lunge position with the right foot forward and left foot back, knee flexed. Shift your weight slightly back, bend the right knee more to feel the stretch in the left calf as you press the left heel toward the floor.

▶ UPPER SHOULDERS AND NECK (TRAPEZIUS): DIAGONAL TILT WITH ROTATION

Sit with your back straight and chest lifted. Lift the right arm diagonally toward the corner of the room. Press the left shoulder down firmly and press your right ear toward the right shoulder (Figure 11-10, *A*).

Increase intensity: Press the head to the side with gentle pressure from the right hand.

Decrease intensity: Press both shoulders downward. Bend the head and neck straight forward to feel a stretch in the rear of the neck and shoulders (Figure 11-10, *B*).

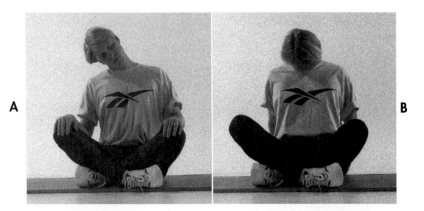

FIGURE 11-10 A, Upper shoulders and neck (trapezius): diagonal tilt with rotation. **B,** To decrease intensity press both shoulders downward. Bend the head and neck straight forward to feel a stretch in the rear of the neck and shoulders.

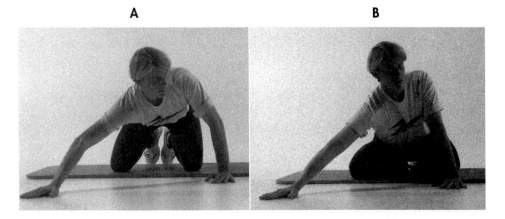

FIGURE 11-11 A, Chest and front shoulders: reach and rotate. **B,** To decrease intensity sit back with buttocks toward heels, right arm straight and out to the side. Rotate torso to the left, twisting from the hip joints and keeping the sternum lifted.

▶ CHEST AND FRONT SHOULDERS: REACH AND ROTATE

Start in the hands-and-knees position with the right arm straight and out to the side. Shift the hips back toward the ankles and turn the torso toward the left to feel a stretch across the right side of the chest and shoulder (Figure 11-11, *A*). Hold the stretch for three to five breaths. Repeat on the left side.

Increase intensity: Same as base action with the right hand on a platform.

Decrease intensity: Sit back with your buttocks toward your heels, right arm straight and out to the side. Rotate your torso to the left, twisting from the hip joints and keeping sternum lifted (Figure 11-11, *B*).

A   B

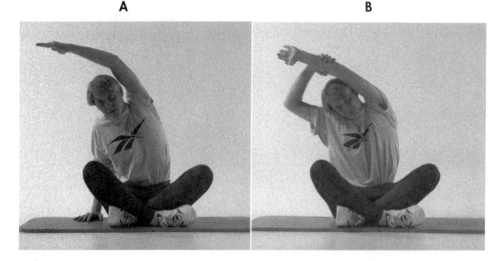

FIGURE 11-12 **A,** Lateral torso (latissimus): hip and rib separation. **B,** To decrease intensity sit with legs crossed, with the left arm lifted. Use the right hand to press the upper arm backward until you feel a stretch along the rear and side of the torso. Be sure not to arch your back.

▶ LATERAL TORSO (LATISSIMUS): HIP AND RIB SEPARATION

Sit with your legs crossed in front and both rear hip bones firmly in contact with the floor. Raise the left arm overhead and lean the torso to the right, supporting the upper body with the right hand. Reach toward the side wall and rotate the torso slightly to feel a stretch along the left side and rear of the torso (Figure 11-12, A). Hold the stretch for three to five breaths.

Increase intensity: Same initial position, but reach farther and rotate the left arm so that the thumb points toward the ceiling.

Decrease intensity: Sit as before with your legs crossed and with the left arm lifted. Use the right hand to press the upper arm backward until you feel a stretch along the rear and side of the torso (Figure 11-12, B). Take care not to allow the back to arch.

▶ SHOULDER ROTATORS: TOWEL STRETCH

Place a towel vertically along the spine, grasping it with both hands as shown. Use the right hand to pull the towel up, stretching the left rotators. Use the left hand to pull the towel down to stretch the right rotators (Figure 11-13, A). Reverse the arm positions and repeat.

Increase intensity: Same position as the base action; grasp the towel with the hands closer together or without a towel, interlocking your fingers (Figure 11-13, B).

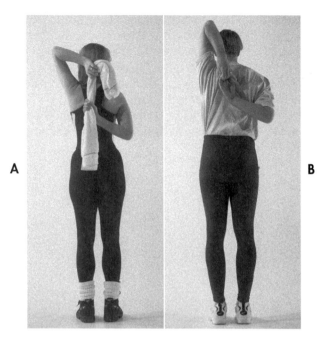

FIGURE 11-13 **A**, Shoulder rotators: towel stretch. **B**, To increase intensity grasp the towel with the hands closer together or without a towel, interlocking fingers.

Decrease intensity: Same position as the base action, grasping the towel with the hands farther apart.

SUMMARY

- Flexibility must be an integral part of a balanced fitness program. As body alignment and muscle balance improve, the chance of acute injury in sports and other activities decreases. Also, the benefit of strength training may be enhanced by allowing movement through a complete range of motion.
- Balanced flexibility is crucial for proper body alignment, which affects not only how you look and feel (physically and emotionally) but also how you are perceived by others.
- Serious flexibility training is performed with the goal in mind of making permanent changes in the length of your connective tissues that will remain after the training session.
- The five principles to increase flexibility are: (1) the tissues must be warm, (2) the stretch must be of low intensity and long duration (sensation of stretch for 30 to 60 seconds), (3) you should contract the muscle opposite the group being

stretched to further relax the muscle group being stretched, (4) you should stretch with the torso in neutral position, and (5) you should stretch daily.

- Stretching is most effective (and safe to do) every day. Part of your action plan should be to stretch daily, even on days you do not take class.
- Some body areas will need more attention than others. Focus on areas of tightness (as determined in Assessments 3-7 to 3-10).
- It is normal that your level of flexibility may vary slightly from day to day depending on your level of stress, hydration level, or the amount of previous day's activities.

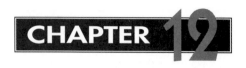

CHAPTER 12

YOUR ACTION PLAN:
MUSCULAR STRENGTH AND ENDURANCE TECHNIQUE AND PROGRESSIONS

OBJECTIVES

After reading this chapter, you should be able to do the following:

- Understand the context of muscular work in an aerobics class as it is applied to increasing muscular strength and endurance.
- Know what type of muscle fibers you are using and which ones to focus on as you train for increased muscular strength or endurance.
- Apply the guidelines for elastic-resistance training to keep your workout safe and effective.
- Effectively perform a range of strength training exercises that focus on developing the muscles of your torso, lower body and upper body.
- Safely increase or decrease the intensity of these exercises to accommodate your level of fitness.

KEY TERMS

While reading this chapter, you will become familiar with the following terms:

► Fast-Twitch Muscle Fibers   ► Slow-Twitch Muscle Fibers
► Postural Muscles

167

MUSCULAR BALANCE AND IMBALANCES

Muscular work in the context of an aerobics class is for the purpose of building both muscular endurance and strength. It is important to build strength and endurance of the muscles that hold the body in safe, neutral alignment, as well as the muscles that move the joints and lift external objects.

To look your best and to prevent injury and undue fatigue, muscle strength must be balanced around each joint. It is important to participate in a program of balanced strength and flexibility training that addresses all the muscle groups.

MUSCULAR IMBALANCES

▶ UPPER BODY IMBALANCES

Pay particular attention to your own muscle imbalances. (See Assessments, Chapter 3.) Poor sitting posture most of the day pulls the torso forward, often overstretching the muscles in the middle back and shoulders and tightening the muscles in the front of the chest and shoulders. Most dance-exercise routines also use the muscles in the front of the chest and arms during the aerobic workout. For better balance, spend time stretching the front muscles and strengthening (not further stretching) the muscles of the upper back, shoulders, and shoulder girdle.

▶ LOWER BODY IMBALANCES

Certain lower body imbalances also develop from long-term sitting positions. A well-rounded program also seeks to create muscle balance in the lower part of the body, particularly with adequate stretching of the hips and calf muscles and by strengthening the muscle groups in the same way they are used from day to day, with compound movements in weight-bearing positions, such as squats and lunges.

OVERLOAD AND TYPES OF RESISTANCE

The amount of overload used during exercise determines whether you are building muscle strength or endurance. Heavier loads (resistance) causing fatigue in 8 to 12 repetitions promote muscle strength. Loads (resistance) causing fatigue in 12 to 20 repetitions promote muscular endurance. Endurance of certain **postural muscles** (such as abdominals and back extensors) is developed through stabilizing exercises, by holding a position over time against outside resistance rather than by performing repetitions of a movement.

Resistance can be applied by various methods. Strength development occurs in response to the intensity of the overload. Muscles do not care what they are working against: they change and grow by having to create internal force. In a dance-exercise class, the resistance for strength development is usually provided by weights, rubber bands, elastic tubing, or body weight. In the gym, machines with pulleys, springs, or hydraulics may also provide the overload for strength development. Each method has its own benefits and limitations. If possible, it is a good idea to train with various tools to receive the benefits of all.

SAFETY GUIDELINES FOR STRENGTH TRAINING EXERCISES

Muscles are composed primarily of two types of muscle fibers, slow-twitch and fast-twitch. The **slow-twitch muscle fibers** are the first fibers called into action in normal low resistance activities such as aerobics or lifting light weights. As the amount of resistance increases—as with heavier weights—the slow-twitch fibers cannot handle the overload alone. Then the **fast-twitch muscle fibers** are recruited to help. Strength training occurs with resistance great enough to recruit the fast-twitch fibers. You know you are working fast-twitch fibers if fatigue occurs after 8 to 12 repetitions, because fast-twitch fibers fatigue quickly. If you can perform more than 12 repetitions you are training the slow-twitch (endurance) fibers, which fatigue slowly

In strength training, the individual muscles are required to create large amounts of force over a shorter period of time, so energy must be created much faster. Because of the different demands in strength training, you must be sure that the body is prepared for this specialized training. The accompanying box provides a list of specific safety guidelines for strength training in which you will be using heavier loads to fatigue the muscles.

▶ **Postural Muscles**

The abdominals and back muscles that are responsible for keeping your body in the neutral position. They can be developed through stabilizing exercises that hold a position, over time, against outside resistance.

▶ **Slow-Twitch Muscle Fibers**

Fairly resistant to fatigue, these are the muscle fibers that are called into action in normal endurance building, low resistance activities such as aerobics or lifting light weights.

▶ **Fast-Twitch Muscle Fibers**

More susceptible to fatigue, these muscle fibers come into play as the amount of resistance increases. They help handle overload and should be the focus of your workout if you are intending to build muscular strength.

Safety Guidelines for Heavy Load Strength Training

1. **Adequate Warm-up.** Warm up adequately before overloading a muscle group for strength training. Because strength-training exercises usually follow the aerobic section of a dance-exercise class, a separate warm-up may not be required. If you are performing strength-training outside of class, however, perform at least one set of 8 to 12 repetitions with little or no resistance, so you can rehearse proper form and stimulate blood delivery to the area.

2. **Slow Controlled Movement.** Perform each exercise slowly with control, taking approximately 2 seconds to complete the up-phase of the movement, and 4 seconds to return to the start position.

3. **Deep, Rhythmical Breathing.** Breathe deeply and rhythmically throughout each exercise. Do not hold your breath.

4. **Precise Technique.** Be very precise with the exercise technique. Pay attention that your torso and joints stay in safe alignment. Do not cheat! Precision, not the amount of weight lifted, should be the primary concern. Poor technique and muscle substitution can cause injury and give a false impression of strength that does not exist.

5. **Use Muscular Control, Not Momentum.** Do not use swinging or flinging movements (momentum) to lift a weight that is too heavy. It is a form of cheating. Joints and connective tissue can be damaged by having to resist high forces not under muscular control. Also do not lock the joints at the end of the range of motion. Make the muscles do the work. If necessary, use less weight to complete the range of motion with perfect form.

6. **Use Enough Resistance to Achieve Muscle Fatigue.** Choose the appropriate resistance to fatigue the targeted muscle group in 8 to 12 repetitions. If the resistance is too light, no strength gains will occur. Repetitions 11 and 12 should be difficult to perform, indicating fatigue of the fast-twitch fibers. Use more resistance if the twelfth repetition is easy. Stop the set or lower the resistance if your technique changes to complete the last few repetitions.

SAFETY GUIDELINES FOR ELASTIC RESISTANCE

Elastic resistance is a convenient and practical method of providing muscular overload when varying sets of weights are not available in a class setting. Elastic provides variable resistance during the exercise movement. As the band stretches, it gets tighter, giving more overload toward the end of the range of motion. Because of the qualities of elastic, sometimes movement techniques will differ from those used when weights are the resistance.

Safety Guidelines for Elastic-Resistance Training

1. Use bands or tubes developed specifically for strength training.
2. Check your tube before each use for small holes or signs of cracking or wear. Do not use a defective tube.
3. Keep your hand and wrist in neutral alignment when holding the band or tube. Your hand and forearm should form a straight line. (See Figure 5-15.)
4. Maintain all nonmoving joints in neutral alignment. Make sure the resistance is delivered to the targeted muscle group, not spread out among several.
5. Control the band throughout the exercise; do not let the tension in the band pull you back to the start position. Resist the tension through the full range of motion: 2 seconds up, 4 seconds to return to start position.
6. Do not use elastic resistance close to your eyes or face. (See Figures 5-20 and 5-21.)
7. Choose the appropriate overload to be able to complete the desired repetitions through the full range of motion. Thicker bands give heavy resistance; thinner ones provide light resistance.
8. You should not feel joint pain during an exercise with elastic resistance. If you do, choose a band with lower resistance or discontinue the exercise.

Besides convenience, elastic resistance provides an advantage of training the muscles that anchor the band as well as the ones that move the band. Be sure that the stabilizing joints and muscles maintain safe, neutral alignment throughout the motion. (See Figures 5-11, 5-12, and 5-14 for a reminder of what incorrect, hyperextended form looks like.)

Take care to follow the safety guidelines in the accompanying box when you are using elastic to overload muscles for strength and endurance.

EXERCISE TECHNIQUE AND PROGRESSION FOR STRENGTH AND ENDURANCE

Figure 8-14 shows the major muscle groups of the body that need to be addressed in a well-rounded strength-training program.

Your instructor will use a wide variety of exercises in class; various exercises will use dumbbells, elastic, or body weight as the overload.

The rest of this chapter will describe three or four exercises each for the upper and lower parts of the body. These are primarily compound movements that use many muscle groups. It is important to master proper execution of each exercise without external resistance first. Remember that form is more important than the amount of weight you use.

Similar to the previous chapters on aerobic and flexibility techniques and progressions, the following section shows strength-training exercises, with ways to increase or decrease the intensity. For each exercise, pay attention to the action and alignment cues that accompany each picture. These cues may be used by your instructor in class. Mastery of proper execution and the fundamentals of movement is important to achieving strength and endurance gains without injury.

Increase intensity by increasing the amount of overload or moving the resistance farther from the moving joint. Decrease the intensity by decreasing the overload or moving the resistance closer to the moving joint. Intensity may also increase if you perform the repetitions more slowly, so that the muscle must contract for a longer period of time. If you perform multiple sets, you can also increase intensity by decreasing the amount of recovery time between sets.

EXERCISES FOR THE TORSO

▶ PELVIC TILTS

This exercise promotes awareness of the abdominal muscles and of the ability to control the position of the pelvis and lower back. It improves proper isolation of the abdominal muscles so that the torso is safely stabilized during upper and lower body strength-training exercises. During strength-training exercises, the abdominals should hold the torso in a neutral position. Neutral position of the pelvis and torso (Figure 12-1) is midway between the forward-tilted position (Figure 12-2, A) and the backward-tilted position (Figure 12-2, B). This exercise goes through the full range of motion, but neither of the extremes of the range are to be maintained or used as a rest position. The torso should be aligned in neutral during relaxed sitting and standing. The stabilization exercises hold the torso in neutral while the legs are moving.

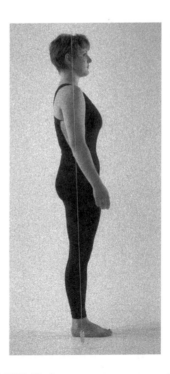

FIGURE 12-1 Neutral position of the pelvis and torso.

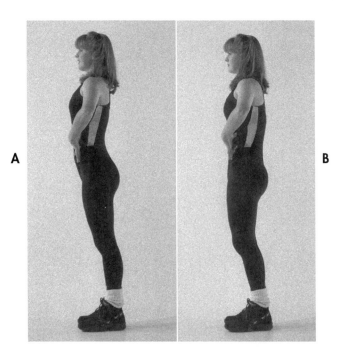

FIGURE 12-2 A, Forward tilt position of pelvis and torso. **B,** Backward tilt position of the pelvis.

Start.   Stand with feet hip-width apart, knees slightly bent, hands on your hips, thumbs on your lower back. Your tail-bone is pointing toward the back wall. Your pelvis is in a forward-tilt.

Action.   Slowly contract your abdominal muscles so that your pelvis rocks back and downward. If your pelvis were a bucket, it would be like pouring water out behind you. Your tailbone points toward the floor between your feet. Your chest stays lifted. Your buttocks stay relaxed.

To return to start, slowly release your abdominal muscles so that your pelvis rocks forward and the tailbone points toward the back wall.

▶ TORSO STABILIZATION, STANDING

This exercise trains your abdominal muscles to hold the torso in safe alignment, even when outside resistance (leg movement and elastic resistance) tries to pull it out of alignment. The elastic tubing provides resistance to the hip extensors (gluteals and hamstrings). The strong hip-muscle contraction tends to pull the torso out of the neutral position. Therefore the abdominal muscles must work intensely to hold the torso in neutral.

Start.   Place a circle of elastic tubing around the ankles. Stand with your weight on the left leg, right leg behind, knee straight, toes resting on the floor. Use the abdominal muscles to hold the torso still in the neutral position (Figure 12-3, *A*).

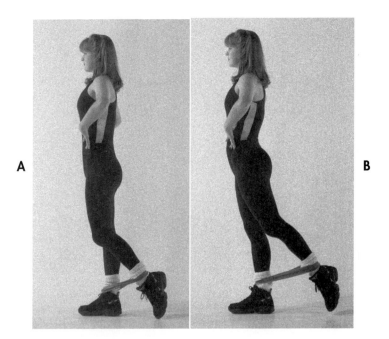

FIGURE 12-3 **A,** Torso stabilization, standing (start position). **B,** Action.

Action. Lift your back leg from the floor (1 or 2 inches) by extending the hip. Keep the torso in *exactly* the same position as the start position (neutral). Keep both front hip bones parallel, facing forward. Do *not* allow the lower back to arch as you lift the back leg (Figure 12-3, *B*)—stabilize the torso with the abdominal muscles.

- Return to start by lowering the rear leg.
- Repeat for 8 to 12 repetitions.
- Repeat with the right leg forward, left behind.

To increase resistance: Bend the back knee to set the elastic at a higher level of tension.

To decrease resistance: Perform without elastic resistance.

▶ TORSO STABILIZATION, LYING FACE UP

The last exercise trained the torso muscles to hold (stabilize) neutral position of the spine when one leg was moving. This exercise trains the abdominal and back muscles to coordinate and stabilize the torso when both legs are moving. The leg movement will tend to pull the back off the floor; the abdominal muscles must work to hold the back flat on the floor against the increasing resistance of the feet moving away from the buttocks.

Start. Lie face up on the floor with the knees and arms overhead. Use your abdominals to press the back flat on the floor (Figure 12-4, *A*). Throughout the

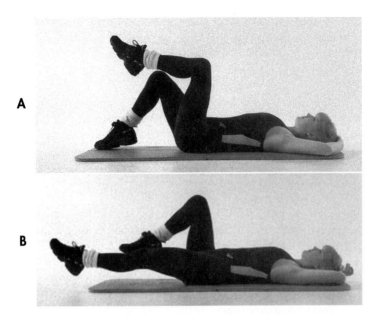

FIGURE 12-4 **A,** Torso stabilization, alternate toe tap. **B,** To increase resistance, place arms overhead and slowly press heels away from torso: focus on keeping back flat.

exercise, focus on the abdominal contraction and on keeping the back flat on the floor. Breathe deeply and rhythmically throughout the sequence.

Action. Use a strong contraction of the abdominal muscles to keep the lower back flat on the floor as you alternate tapping the right foot then the left foot to the floor.

- Repeat for 8 to 12 alternating sets (right then left is one set).

To increase resistance: Place both arms overhead, and alternate pressing right then left foot away from the torso (Figure 12-4, *B*).

To decrease resistance: Tap only your toes to the floor, placing your arms by your sides.

▶ TORSO CURLS WITH ACTIVE TILT

This exercise combines contraction of several abdominal muscles to press the back flat and curl the upper torso forward. The feet are placed away from the buttocks to provide resistance for the oblique abdominals, pressing the back flat and the pelvis backward (this exercise is illustrated in Figure 8-5).

Start. Lie face up on the floor with the knees slightly bent and the heels on the floor away from the buttocks. Arms are crossed on the chest. There will be a space between your lower back and the floor.

Action. Go through the routine in the following 4-step progression:

- (1) **Tilt:** Use your abdominal muscles to tilt the pelvis back and press the lower back flat to the floor.

- (2) **Curl:** With your back flat, curl your head and shoulders forward until the shoulder blades lift off the floor.
- (3) **Uncurl:** Lower the head and shoulders to the floor.
- (4) **Untilt:** Release the lower abdominals to allow the lower back to raise off the floor.
- Repeat the tilt and curl sequence 8 to 12 times.

To increase resistance: Place your arms overhead. (See Figure 8-8.)

To decrease resistance: Place your arms flat, 45 degrees out to the side, elbows straight, palms up. (See Figure 8-4.)

▶ TORSO EXTENSION

This exercise equalizes and strengthens the muscles on either side of your spine. Focus on different regions of your back by lifting various parts (head and shoulders only; head, shoulders, and upper chest; head, shoulders, and rib cage).

Start.　Lie on the floor, face down, arms by your side. Squeeze your buttocks and hold the hip bones in contact with the floor (Figure 12-5, *A*).

Action.　Lift the upper torso (head and shoulders, or head, shoulders, and chest; or head, shoulders, and rib cage) from the floor.

- Slowly lower the upper torso to the floor.
- Repeat for 8 to 12 repetitions.

To increase resistance: Place the hands on the shoulders (Figure 12-5, *B*).

To decrease resistance: Place the hands on the floor beneath the shoulders to assist with the torso movement.

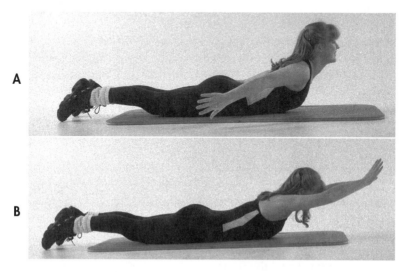

FIGURE 12-5　A, Torso extension: lift upper torso from the floor. **B,** To increase resistance lift arms overhead.

EXERCISES FOR THE UPPER BODY

▶ BENT-OVER ROWS WITH WEIGHTS

This exercise trains the spinal muscles to hold safe alignment against resistance. It also strengthens the muscles of the upper back and shoulder blades. It can be used in combination with elbow curls or elbow extensions to strengthen the biceps or triceps. Be sure to keep the back muscles contracted with a slight downward arch of the lower back throughout the exercise.

Start.   Stand with your feet hip-width apart, knees and hips bent. The torso is held diagonally to the floor with the abdominal and back muscles co-contracted and a slight downward arch at the lower back. The tailbone and the chest are lifted. Arms are held away from the sides, elbows bent and hands in line with the knees, holding weights with a relaxed grip (Figure 12-6, *A*).

Action.   Squeeze the shoulder blades together, then pull the elbows toward each other. The hands will follow; do not use the biceps to lift the hands. Keep the shoulders down; do not shrug (Figure 12-6, *B*). Return to the start position. Repeat for 8 to 12 repetitions.

To increase resistance: Use heavier weights.

To decrease resistance: Use no weights.

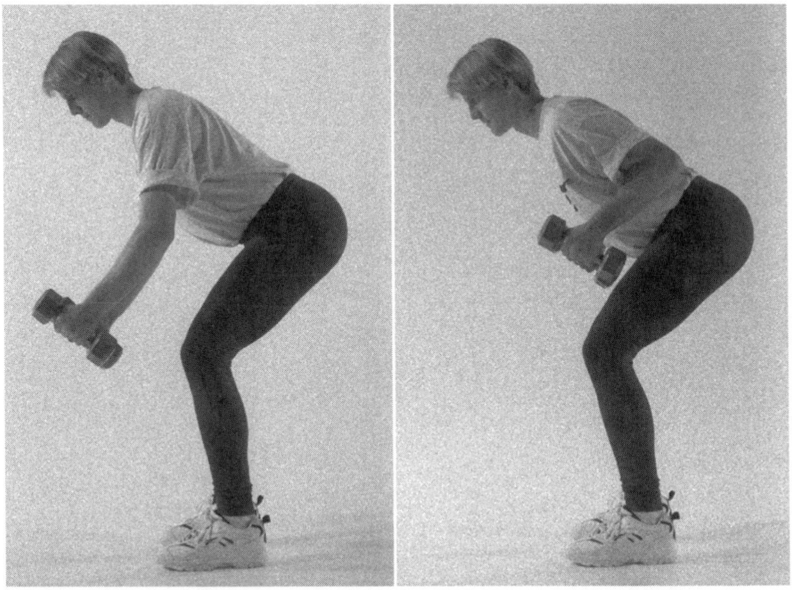

FIGURE 12-6   Bent-over rows with weights. **A,** Start position. **B,** Action.

▶ **OVERHEAD PRESS**

This exercise trains the shoulder muscles to coordinate properly with each other and strengthens the deltoids, upper pectorals, and triceps. Be sure to use your abdominal muscles to hold your torso stable (prevent the back from arching) as the arms lift overhead. Then the movement trains the torso as well as the arms and shoulders.

Start.   Sit upright without external support, with elastic anchored under the feet. Keep wrists neutral, starting with hands at shoulder level (Figure 12-7, *A*).

Action.   Press your hands upward and slightly forward. Straighten the elbows as the arms press upward (Figure 12-7, *B*).

To increase resistance: Use dumbbells (Figure 12-7, *C*).

To decrease resistance: Use no weight.

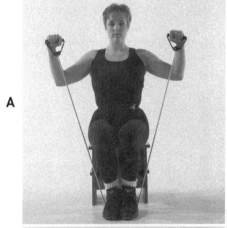

A

FIGURE 12-7   Overhead press. **A,** Start position. **B,** Action— press hands upward and slightly forward. **C,** To increase resistance use dumbbells.

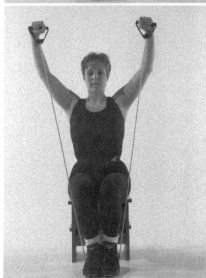

B

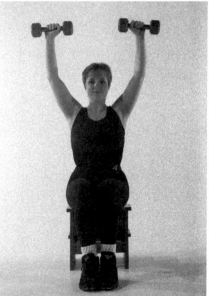

C

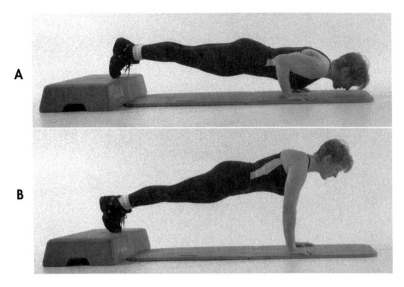

FIGURE 12-8 Push-ups with increased resistance. **A,** Start position. **B,** Action.

▶ PUSH-UPS

This old standby is an important strengthener of the chest and arms. If performed properly, it also trains the muscles of the neck and torso to prevent the torso from sagging and the head from dropping. Hold the head, back, and torso straight in line with the legs throughout the movement.

Start.   Lie face down, with the hands beneath the shoulders. Hold the body in a straight line. (See Figure 3-17.)

Action.   Press the floor away with your hands, lifting the body as a rigid bar, until the elbows are straight.

- Slowly lower the straight torso toward the floor to return to start.
- Do not allow the head or lower back to drop or sag.
- Repeat for 8-12 repetitions.

To increase resistance: Place your feet on a step (Figure 12-8, *A* and *B*).

To decrease resistance: Push up from your knees rather than your toes. Bend your knees so that your weight is on the lower thigh area, above the kneecaps. (See Figure 3-18.)

EXERCISES FOR THE LOWER BODY

▶ SQUAT

This exercise trains the lower body and entire torso to lift objects safely from the floor. The muscles that lift are the knee extensors (quadriceps) and the hip extensors (gluteals and hamstrings). The muscles that stabilize the torso are the

A   B   C

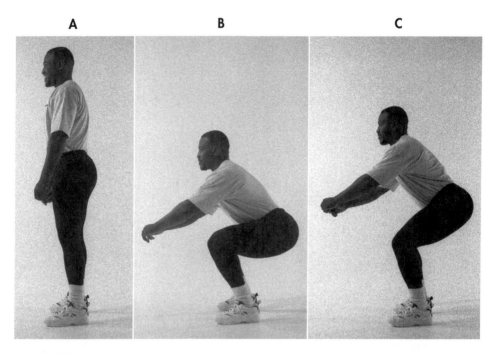

FIGURE 12-9 Squat. **A,** Start position. **B,** Action. **C,** To decrease intensity, use a smaller range of motion with less bend at the hips and knees.

abdominals, particularly the obliques, and the spinal extensors. The torso muscles contract isometrically to hold the torso in safe alignment. The arm muscles must also contract isometrically to grip the weights or other object to be lifted.

Start.   Stand upright with your feet shoulder-width apart and parallel or slightly turned out. Your spine should be aligned so that there is a slight inward curve at the lower back. The tailbone is pointed toward the floor slightly behind your feet. The chest is lifted (Figure 12-9, *A*).

Action.   Follow this procedure:
- Sit as far back as possible.
- Think of touching the back wall with your hips.
- Keep your heels on the floor.
- Keep your body weight on the entire foot.
- Keep your knees aligned over your feet (ankles).
- Keep your chest lifted.
- Be conscious that your abdominals and back muscles are contracting isometrically to keep your torso stable throughout the motion (Figure 12-9, *B*).

To increase intensity: Hold weights in the hands or perform a lunge (see instructions under the next exercise).

To decrease intensity: Use a smaller range of motion, with less bend at the hips and knees (Figure 12-9, *C*).

A   B   C

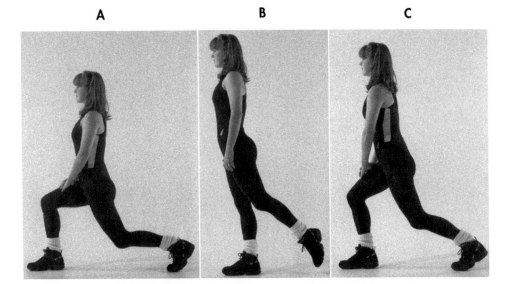

FIGURE 12-10 Stationary lunge. **A,** Start position. **B,** Action. **C,** To decrease intensity, use a smaller range of motion with less bend at the hip and knee or decrease the width of the stance.

▶ STATIONARY LUNGE

This exercise also trains the torso and lower body for lifting activities, and the muscles will be stronger for activities such as hill- or stair-climbing. And, of course, as the muscle function improves the muscle form and shape will also improve. This exercise also targets the hip extensors (gluteus maximus and hamstrings) and the knee extensors (quadriceps) as the squat does, but it also uses the inner and outer muscles of the hip and thigh to stabilize the leg and pelvis. This exercise also stimulates more balance, stabilization, and flexibility of the lower leg and ankle, because the movement is controlled by the front leg only. The torso muscles will also gain endurance as they contract isometrically to hold the torso in safe alignment.

Start. Legs are a large stride-length apart, front to back. Feet are hip-width apart, side-to-side. Toes are forward or slightly turned out. Back heel is lifted (Figure 12-10, *A*).

Action. Bend the front knee and lower front thigh to be parallel with the floor.
- Keep the shin vertical, knee aligned with ankle.
- Keep the chest lifted.
- Keep your body weight on the front foot.
- Return to start by straightening the front knee.
- Do not push with the rear foot.
- Make the front thigh and hip muscles do all the work (Figure 12-10, *B*).

To increase intensity: Hold weights in the hands.

To decrease intensity: Use a smaller range of motion, with less bend at the hip and knee or decrease the width of the stance (Figure 12-10, *C*).

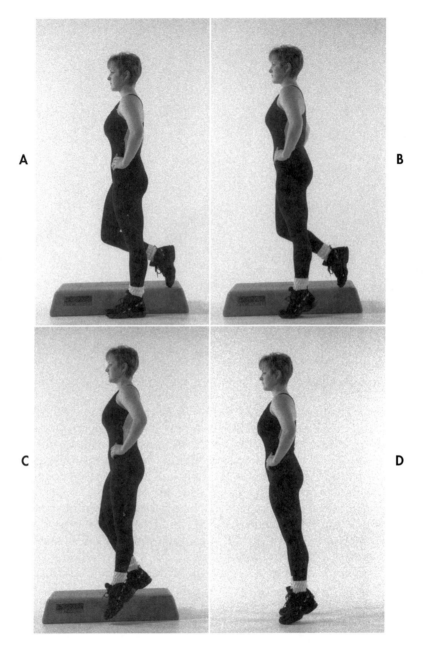

FIGURE12-11 Single heel lifts. **A,** Start position. **B,** Action. **C,** To increase intensity, push the ball of the foot firmly into the floor to lift the body weight off the floor. **D,** To decrease intensity, stand with weight distributed evenly on both feet; lift and lower heels slowly, keeping ankles straight.

▶ HEEL LIFTS

This exercise strengthens the calf muscles and trains balance and the stabilizing muscles of the ankle and foot. Start with double heel lifts, then progress to single heel lifts for more balance work.

Start.   Stand beside a step platform with the right knee bent and toes resting on top of the step. All body weight is on the left foot (Figure 12-11, *A*).

Action.   Lift the left heel slowly (Figure 12-11, *B*); do 8 to 12 repetitions.

To increase intensity: Use the same initial position as in Figure 12-11, *A*, but instead of slowly lifting the left heel, push the ball of the foot firmly into the floor to lift the body weight off the floor (Figure 12- 11, *C*).

To decrease intensity: Stand upright with your weight distributed evenly on both feet. Knees should be straight but not pushed back. Lift and lower your heels slowly, keeping your ankles straight (Figure 12-11, *D*). Do 8 to 12 repetitions. Tailbone should point toward the floor slightly behind the heels. Chest is lifted and arms are lifted to the side, shoulders down.

SUMMARY

- Muscular strength plays an important role in holding your body in neutral alignment and needs to be balanced around each joint.
- Lower body muscle imbalances can develop from spending too much time in a sitting position.
- A well-rounded training program seeks to create muscle balance in the lower body and should be combined with stretching of the hips and calf muscles.
- To safely train with heavier loads, you should perform an adequate warm-up, use slow, controlled movements, maintain a deep, rhythmical breathing pattern, focus on a precise technique, focus on control versus momentum and use enough momentum to achieve muscle fatigue.
- Elastic resistance is an excellent alternative to training with weights and provides variable resistance during the exercise movement. Elastic resistance provides the advantage of training the muscles that anchor the band as well as the ones that move the band.
- You can choose from a number of exercises to increase muscular strength, and aerobic instructors work with a wide range of dumbbell, elastic, or body-weight exercises into their classes to help you achieve overload.
- To maintain muscular balance it is important to focus on muscles of the torso, upper body and lower body.
- While training for strength it is important to pay attention to proper form and complete execution of the action, and to be sure to increase or decrease the intensity of an exercise to accommodate your individual level of fitness.

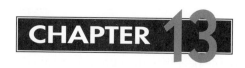

YOUR ACTION PLAN:
A **LIFETIME**
OF **FITNESS**

▽

OBJECTIVES

After reading this chapter, you should be able to do the following:

- Explore the possibilities of cross-training to keep your exercise routine fresh and challenging.
- Choose the activities that you like and that fit with your caloric expenditure needs to vary your workout.

KEY TERM

While reading this chapter, you will become familiar with the following term:

► **Cross-training**

It Up—cont'd

Activity	Cal/hr 100 lb	Cal/hr 125 lb	Cal/hr 150 lb	Cal/hr 175 lb	Cal/hr 200 lb
Lacrosse (game)	384	480	576	672	768
Racquetball (competitive)	480	600	720	840	960
Rock or mountain climbing	384	480	576	672	768
Rope jumping (slow)	384	480	576	672	768
Rope jumping (medium)	480	600	720	840	960
Rope jumping (fast)	576	720	864	1008	1152
Rowing (individual 4-6 mph)	336	420	504	588	672
Rowing (individual >6 mph)	576	720	864	1008	1152
Running (5 mph)	384	480	576	672	768
Running (6 mph)	480	600	720	840	960
Running (7 mph)	552	690	828	966	1104
Running (8 mph)	648	810	972	1134	1296
Running (9 mph)	720	900	1080	1260	1440
Running (10 mph)	768	960	1152	1344	1536
Skateboarding	240	300	360	420	480
Skiing (cross country, 4-5 mph)	384	480	576	672	768
Skiing (cross country, 5-8 mph)	432	540	648	756	864
Skiing (cross country, >8 mph)	672	840	1008	1176	1344
Skiing (downhill)	288	360	432	504	576
Skiing (water)	288	360	432	504	576
Soccer (competitive)	480	600	720	840	960
Stairmaster (level 7)	384	480	576	672	768
Stairmaster (level 9)	480	600	720	840	960
Stairmaster (level 11)	576	720	864	1008	1152
Step aerobics (low intensity)	288	360	432	504	576
Step aerobics (moderate intensity)	384	480	576	672	768
Step aerobics (high intensity)	480	600	720	840	960
Swimming (freestyle, 50 yds/min)	384	480	576	672	768
Swimming (freestyle, 75 yds/min)	528	660	792	924	1056
Tennis (doubles)	288	360	432	504	576
Tennis (singles)	384	480	576	672	768
Volleyball (competitive)	192	240	288	336	384
Walking (2 mph)	144	180	216	252	288
Walking (3 mph)	168	210	252	294	336
Walking (4 mph)	192	240	288	336	384

Continued

IT IS UP TO YOU TO TAKE IT FROM HERE

What will you do once you have finished this course? Our hope is that you will continue to enjoy aerobic dance exercise and that your workouts will be one part of the big picture of a healthy lifestyle. You will be able to use the material covered in this book for the rest of your life as you make dietary and lifestyle choices. Even though you may have come to love aerobic dance exercise, remember that there are many ways to train aerobically—and that aerobic fitness is only one piece of the fitness puzzle!

CONSIDER CROSS-TRAINING FOR OPTIMAL RESULTS

Cross-training, participating in a variety of different fitness activities, has become extremely popular because it is both effective and fun. Cross-training uses the principles of training discussed in Chapter 2 to maximize the return on your time and the energy you spend in any activity. Rather than limiting your workouts to one mode of exercise, cross-training provides a means for your body to adapt specifically to various forms and types of overload. If your workout routine remains the same all the time, your body may become "stale" or unresponsive. By cross-training, you can make each workout a surprise for your body. A well-rounded fitness program benefits tremendously not only from training each of the components of fitness, but also from varying the type of training performed within each component.

THE ACTIVITY PYRAMID

The Activity Pyramid developed by the Park Nicollet Medical Foundation (Figure 13-1) is one way to look at the effect any type of physical activity can have on your overall health and well-being. As with the Food Pyramid, you want to perform the everyday activities forming the base of the pyramid as often as possible. If you look for ways to be active throughout the day, even simple activities such as climbing stairs can become part of your cross-training regimen. Vigorous physical or recreational activity is usually something you need to plan into your schedule, so select activities that you find fun and enjoyable to keep both your interest and participation high. If you incorporate a variety of activities into your plan, chances are your plan will work and you will see results.

▶ **Cross-training**

Participation in a variety of fitness activities; it keeps your workout challenging and fun and provides an excellent way for your body to adapt to various forms of overload.

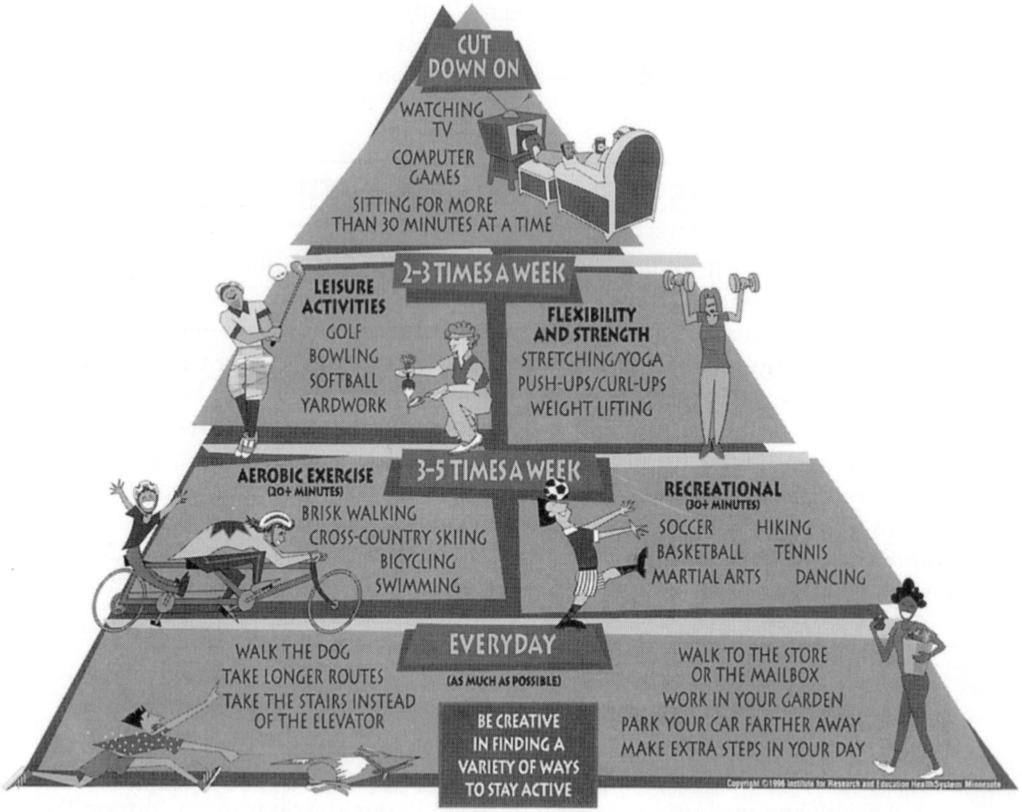

FIGURE 13-1 The Activity Pyramid. If you are starting from a position of little or no physical activity, begin at the bottom of the pyramid and work your way up. Increase your level of activity throughout the day by "doing it yourself" instead of relying on modern conveniences. If you are someone who works out occasionally, focus on the middle of the pyramid. Increase your regular participation in activities that focus on the health-related components of fitness as well as active leisure and recreational activities. If you are at a well-developed level of fitness, you can use this pyramid as a guide to keep your fitness program new and exciting; dedicate yourself to developing a new skill or trying a new activity. (From the Institute for Research and Education, HealthSystem Minnesota. Copyright © 1996. Reprinted with permission.)

CALORIC EXPENDITURE OF SELECT AC[TIVITIES]

Use the accompanying Add It Up chart to compare the pot[ential] caloric expenditures from a variety of activities. Calories burned [are] provided in the journal *Medicine and Science in Sports and Exercis[e]*. [Look] closest to your body weight for the approximate caloric cost. T[his may be] slightly higher or lower, depending on your actual body weight [and whether] you perform the work more or less vigorously.

Add It Up

Activity	Cal/hr 100 lb	Cal/hr 125 lb	Cal/hr 150 lb	Cal/hr 175 [lb]
Aerobic dance (low intensity)	288	360	432	50[4]
Aerobic dance (moderate intensity)	384	480	576	672
Aerobic dance (high intensity)	480	600	720	840
Badminton (doubles)	216	270	324	378
Badminton (competitive singles)	336	420	504	588
Basketball (game)	384	480	576	672
Bicycling (10-12 mph)	288	360	432	504
Bicycling (12-14 mph)	384	480	576	672
Bicycling (14-16 mph)	480	600	720	840
Bicycling (16-19 mph)	576	720	864	1008
Bicycling (>20 mph)	768	960	1152	1344
Dancing (ballroom, slow)	144	180	216	252
Dancing (ballroom, fast)	264	330	396	462
Football (game—touch or flag)	384	480	576	672
Field hockey (game)	384	480	576	672
Golf (using power cart)	168	210	252	294
Golf (using pull cart)	240	300	360	420
Golf (carrying clubs)	264	330	396	462
Handball	576	720	864	1008
Horseback riding (general)	192	240	288	336
Ice hockey (game)	384	480	576	672
Ice skating (<9 mph)	264	330	396	462
Ice skating (>9 mph)	432	540	648	756
Inline skating (12.8 mph)	576	720	864	1008

Continu[ed]

Add It Up—cont'd

Activity	Cal/hr 100 lb	Cal/hr 125 lb	Cal/hr 150 lb	Cal/hr 175 lb	Cal/hr 200 lb
Walking (4.5 mph)	216	270	324	378	432
Walking (4 mph, 5% grade)	336	420	504	588	672
Walking (4 mph, 10% grade)	480	600	720	840	960
Water aerobics (low intensity)	192	240	288	336	384
Water aerobics (moderate intensity)	288	360	432	504	576
Water aerobics (high intensity)	432	540	648	756	864

Adapted from Ainsworth BE, Haskell WL, Leon AS, Jacobs DR Jr, Montoye HJ, Sallis JF, and Paffenbarger RS Jr: Compendium of physical activities: classification of energy costs of human physical activities, Med Sci Sports Exerc. 25:71-80, 1993.

SUMMARY

- Cross-training and looking for ways throughout the day to increase your level of physical activity will make your pursuit of fitness an integral part of your life.
- Aerobic fitness is only one piece of the fitness puzzle. The principles described in this book and a passion for aerobic dance exercise will help you continue to put it all together!

Appendix

HOW TO CHOOSE A QUALITY AEROBIC FITNESS INSTRUCTOR

What makes an exercise class enjoyable and effective? Is it the music, the movements, or the feeling of camaraderie among the students? The factor underlying all these aspects is the instructor. A knowledgeable instructor with a fun personality determines the quality of the class.

The 15 points in this worksheet will help you select a high-quality instructor who will help you make the most of your exercise class.

Yes No

☐ ☐ Is the instructor trained in anatomy, exercise physiology, kinesiology, injury prevention, first aid, and monitoring of exercise? Is she or he certified by a nationally recognized organization such as ACE, ACSM, or a recognized equivalent?

To prepare a class that gives you a safe, effective workout, an instructor needs a good grounding in exercise science and exercise technique. An exercise certification indicates that the instructor has at least basic knowledge in the areas necessary to teach a quality class. You can check with the instructor, fitness director, or facility owner/manager to verify what kind of education, training, and certification the instructor has.

Yes No

☐ ☐ Does the instructor belong to a professional fitness association, such as IDEA or IRSA, to keep current with the latest exercise theories and techniques?

The exercise industry is changing all the time, so it is crucial that an instructor know the latest research to plan a safe class. Membership in a professional fitness association is one way you can tell that an instructor is staying current.

Yes No

☐ ☐ Does the instructor ask about medical conditions and previous injuries that may affect your exercise program?

Many medical conditions can affect your participation in class, and a good instructor will help you make the most of class without compromising your health.

191

Yes No

☐ ☐   Is the instructor certified in cardiopulmonary resuscitation (CPR)?

Exercisers of all ages and ranges of medical backgrounds take group exercise classes. Safety training enables an instructor to know what to do in case of an emergency (e.g., if a student has chest pains) in class.

Yes No

☐ ☐   Does the instructor ask about your current level of fitness? Does the instructor provide modifications of exercises or alternatives for students of varying fitness levels or with special limitations?

An instructor should be able to show moves that are suitable for beginner, intermediate, and advanced participants and those with a variety of health concerns. An instructor should encourage you to go at your own pace and stop and rest if you feel pain or fatigue.

Yes No

☐ ☐   Does the instructor explain the benefits of each exercise and demonstrate how to do each one correctly and in a controlled manner?

Your instructor should let you know which muscles you are working and how to exercise using proper technique. The instructor shouldn't set a pace faster than the majority of the class can keep up with.

Yes No

☐ ☐   Does the instructor explain the importance of heart rate monitoring and perceived exertion and have students check levels during class?

For an effective cardiovascular workout, participants need to exercise at a certain intensity during class. The instructor should either have you take your pulse rate or teach you the perceived exertion scale and ask you to rate your exertion during class.

Yes No

☐ ☐   Does the instructor move around the room to give individual instruction?

A good instructor will move throughout the class at different points to check for proper technique and to get to know participants.

Yes No

☐ ☐   Can the instructor clearly be heard above the music?

Because the movement directions and safety reminders the instructor gives are important, you should be able to hear these above the music. The music used in class should be exciting and motivate you to exercise. The instructor should clearly pronounce words so you can understand them. The instructor should vary his or her vocal tones, not speak in a monotone.

Yes   No

☐   ☐   Does the class move smoothly from one type of exercise to the next?

An exercise class should be well organized. An instructor should not need to stop and think between sections. The music should be prepared, so the instructor doesn't waste class time dealing with it. The class should start with exercises that warm up your body and should end with a cool-down and stretching exercises.

Yes   No

☐   ☐   Does the instructor encourage a noncompetitive atmosphere that allows all participants to work out at their own level?

A caring instructor will make all students feel like winners. You should never feel you have to keep up with more advanced exercisers. All shapes and sizes of exercisers should feel welcome in the class, and all students should be encouraged. The focus of the class should be on exercising to improve or maintain health, not just on working out to look better.

Yes   No

☐   ☐   Is the instructor friendly and interested in you as a person?

Does the instructor make an attempt to learn your name? Do you feel like the instructor really cares about you and your well-being? A good instructor will make an effort to build a one-on-one relationship with regular students.

Yes   No

☐   ☐   Does the instructor interact with the students most of the time or does he or she look into the mirror more frequently?

A good instructor will be interested in what you are doing, not in his or her own movements. Look for an instructor who maintains eye contact with different people throughout the class. An instructor should never put his or her own workout before helping you have an effective, safe, enjoyable class.

Yes   No

☐   ☐   Will the instructor answer questions before or after class?

A qualified instructor will be happy to explain moves you don't understand. He or she should be eager to share health and fitness knowledge with you and provide advice on how you can improve your fitness level in class.

Yes   No

☐   ☐   Does the instructor create a fun atmosphere?

You may be able to answer "yes" to all of the above questions, but if you don't have fun in class, you probably won't stick with it long. Although instructors don't have to be stand-up comedians, their enthusiastic personality and manner should help you enjoy the class.

Reprinted by permission from IDEA, the International Association of Fitness Professionals, (800) 999-IDEA; (619) 535-8779, ext. 7.

REFERENCES

American College of Sports Medicine Position Stand: The recommended quantity and quality of exercise for developing and maintaining cardiorespiratory and muscular fitness in healthy adults, Medicine and Science in Sports and Exercise, 22:265–274, 1990.

American College of Sports Medicine Position Stand: Proper and improper weight–loss programs, Medicine and Science in Sports and Exercise, 15:ix–xiii, 1983.

Golding LA, Myers CR, Sinning WE, editors: The Y's way to physical fitness: the complete guide to fitness testing and instruction, ed. 3, 1989, Human Kinetics Publishers, Inc.

Fox EL and Mathews DK: Interval training: conditioning for sports and general fitness. Philadelphia, 1974, W.B. Saunders Co.

INDEX